Next Generation NCLEX-RN Study Guide

2024-2025

Complete Review + 600 Test Questions and Detailed Answer Explanations (4 Full-Length Exams)

Table of Contents

Introduction

Nursing care all over the world continues to evolve. With new research and modern tools, nursing care delivery is beginning to realize its fullest potential. But with the advancement in technology and devices to enhance care comes a rise in expectations and demands to deliver an ever-increasing quality of care. This is why nursing councils and boards revise and continually raise their standards for nursing licensing exams.

This guide includes 600 practice questions with explanations and theory material to explain the most important concepts relevant to the NCLEX examination.

How to Make the Most of This Guide

1. A minimum of six hours of study every week is recommended, with three to four hours studying the content material and two to three hours studying past questions.

2. Simulate examination conditions while answering the test questions, which are similar to the questions that will appear on the NCLEX-RN examination.

3. Work with friends and teams to prepare for the examination. This has been shown to be effective in helping memory retention.

Happy studying.

Exam Information

The National Council Licensure Examination (NCLEX) examination is a licensing examination used to test nurses and determine their eligibility to practice in the United States.

The NCLEX-RN examination is for graduates with an associate degree in nursing (ADN) or a bachelor of science in nursing (BSN).

NCLEX Registration

1. All candidates are required to register for their professional nursing license with the state board where they intend to obtain their license.

2. Candidates must meet all the eligibility requirements of the state where they are registered to take the NCLEX-RN examinations.

3. The official testing company for the examinations is Pearson VUE, and all candidates must register with the company.

4. Successful candidates will receive an acknowledgment email from Pearson VUE once the state board confirms their eligibility to take the exams.

5. After confirmation and payment, candidates may schedule the date and time of their examination.

Terminology

The following is a list of some of the terminology used in the examinations:

- **Client:** Refers to patients. Both patient and client may be used interchangeably.
- **Groups:** Refers to two or more clients or patients.
- **Prescription:** An order, intervention, remedy, or treatment plan that is prescribed by an authorized healthcare giver.
- **Exhibit:** Refers to pictures, diagrams, charts, or records.

- **Unlicensed Assistive Personnel (UAP):** Any unlicensed healthcare personnel who can function in a supportive role to nurses and can perform delegated tasks.

Rules and Regulations

Candidates may NOT do any of the following:

- Attempt the examination for someone else.
- Render or receive any form of assistance during the examination.
- Utilize any form of prohibited aids, such as cell phones or smart watches.
- Create any form of disturbance.
- Tamper with the computer systems used for the examination.

If any of these rules are violated, candidates risk dismissal or cancellation of results. They are also at risk of disqualification from future NCLEX examinations.

The NCLEX-RN examination is divided into four main categories:

1. Safe and effective care environment, which is divided into the following:

    a. Management of care.

    b. Safety and infection control.

2. Health promotion and maintenance.

3. Psychosocial integrity.

4. Physiological integrity, which is divided into the following:

    a. Basic care and comfort.

    b. Pharmacological and parenteral therapies.

    c. Reduction of risk potential.

    d. Physiological adaptation.

Chapter 1: Safe and Effective Care Environment

A safe setting is required for the delivery of quality healthcare. That is, a safe environment for both the clients and the healthcare personnel.

Safety in this context includes but is not limited to physical safety. For nurses, this also extends to providing quality and essential information to clients during the process of health delivery. To achieve a safe and effective care environment, nurses must master the management of care and safety and infection control.

Management of Care

Management of care involves the provision and coordination of nursing care in such a way that the delivery of healthcare is safer for both the clients and the healthcare personnel. It entails the following components.

Advance Directives

This term refers to legal documentation that clearly states the wishes of patients about their care should they become unable to communicate. There are several documents for this, and they include the following:

1. **Living will:** This is a document that usually contains a list of the types of treatments and healthcare interventions that individuals do or do not want should they no longer be able to give informed consent. It should be as specific as possible. If a particular intervention or treatment is not listed in the living will, the responsibility falls to the healthcare proxy to make the decision. Some commonly listed interventions include CPR, invasive procedures, surgery, and nasogastric intubation.
2. **Healthcare proxy/ durable power of attorney for healthcare:** This document names an individual with the right to make decisions concerning healthcare when the patient is incapacitated.
3. **Uniform Anatomical Gift Act**: In the U.S., this act allows individuals who are alive to indicate their willingness to donate their organs or tissues upon their death. It also allows relatives of a deceased individual to decide to donate an organ if that individual did not make the decision while alive. It

includes several regulations that prevent the sale or trafficking of human body parts.

Integrating Advance Directives into Clients' Plans of Care

In informing or educating patients about advance directives, patients must be told about self-determination.

Congress passed the Patient Self-Determination Act in 1990. It requires healthcare facilities to inform patients of their rights to make decisions about their care, including the right to accept or refuse treatment and the right to have advance directives.

If an individual already has prepared advance directives, the nurse should document this in the patient's records. If the patient does not have advance directions, the individual should be educated and then allowed to make choices. Copies of patients' advance directives must be placed in their charts.

The most important thing about advance directives is to ensure they are carried out as the occasion demands. The nurse must counsel the patient, family members, and members of staff who might not be familiar with advance directives.

In integrating advance directives with client care, an important document is the five wishes. The five wishes document tells health professionals and relatives the following:

- The individual who will make decisions when a patient cannot.
- The types of medical interventions that a patient accepts or rejects.
- How comfortable the patient wants to be during care.
- How the patient wants to be treated.
- What the patient wants loved ones to know.

Another document that can be useful in clients' decision-making in healthcare is the value history. This document describes the beliefs, opinions, and principles of the client. Although it is not a legal document, it is useful in determining some decisions regarding how a patient is handled and how individuals' beliefs will affect their treatment and care.

Advocacy

Nurses are trained to be advocates for their patients. This means that when decisions are to be made for their clients, they should have the best interests of their clients at heart. Advocacy in this sense can take different forms. It might involve extensive education and sensitization of patients and families. It might also involve explaining diagnoses, tests, or examination findings to the patients and their families. Advocacy from nurses can also involve ensuring that the plan of care is carried out safely and at the right time. Other times, advocacy can involve seeking help from other healthcare professionals and non-medical workers, such as spiritual advisors or social workers.

In all, the goal of advocacy is to speak on behalf of patients and always defend their rights and interests. Advocacy involves the following elements:

1. **Being present:** Advocacy cannot happen if the nurse is absent, especially at times that matter most. Patients spend more time with nurses and as such, open up more easily when it comes to discussing their concerns with them. Then, registered nurses (RNs) can discuss matters with doctors or other healthcare workers.
2. **Listening to patients:** RNs must be patient enough to listen to the concerns and complaints of patients, even when they are not entirely correct. RNs should also pay attention to nonverbal communication. Patients might not be comfortable with the medications or interventions being prescribed. However, they might not voice their worry, and an observant nurse must be aware of nonverbal cues to be able to address the concerns.
3. **Discussion of specified treatment modalities with the clients and respect for whatever decisions they make:** Treatment options should be discussed in detail with patients. Patients who understand an intervention usually cooperate more with the healthcare team. Therefore, the first step of advocacy is educating the clients. In doing this, the nurse should ensure that simple terms are used so that the client understands fully. Some of the things to be discussed include the treatment itself, the procedure, benefits, possible risks and side effects, personnel carrying out the procedure, and alternatives to the procedure.

4. **Advocacy to staff members:** Advocacy requires updating other nursing staff members about client advocacy and how this role should be seamlessly integrated into their practice. Other information that should be provided includes the right of clients to make decisions on their healthcare, which includes accepting or rejecting medical interventions. Advocacy to other staff members should include documenting or orally communicating the client's needs to other staff members, as well as utilizing advocacy resources efficiently. For instance, this might involve getting an interpreter when a patient does not communicate in the nurse's language. It can also involve employing external resources, for instance, occupational therapists, who are non-medical healthcare team members.

Delegation

In the nursing profession, delegation means a nurse transfers a responsibility or task to another nursing staff member but still retains responsibility for the outcome of the task.

To help in the appropriate delegation of responsibilities, the American Nurses Association (ANA) has created the Five Rights of Delegation.

These rights are five areas that must be clearly addressed when assigning care to other staff. They include the following:

- The right person.
- The right task.
- The right circumstances.
- The right direction/communication.
- The right supervision/evaluation.

The Right Task

Is this a task to be delegated?

Not all tasks can or should be delegated. The nature of the task will determine if it can be delegated. Some tasks involve meeting the needs of clients who are in dynamic or unstable conditions. Here, there can be rapid changes that require quick judgment calls and higher competence. Such tasks should not be delegated.

The Right Person

Is this person right for the task?

An RN must assign jobs based on people's skills and knowledge. A licensed practical nurse (LPN) can be assigned tasks that involve a stable patient. Nursing assistants can be assigned tasks that have to do with the maintenance of basic hygiene. Assigning a task to the wrong professional can be dangerous and should be avoided.

The Right Circumstances

What is the state of the patient?

Is the patient stable or unstable? An RN should handle the care of an unstable patient. If the patient becomes stable, then the RN can delegate the task after confirming that the circumstances have changed.

The Right Communication

Is there a clear and detailed explanation of the task to be performed?

A task must be clearly spelled out if it is to be delegated.

The Right Supervision

Who will be held accountable for the outcome of this task?

Responsibility and accountability are key in the nursing profession. Suppose an RN is assigned a supervisory role. This means the RN oversees members of the team, such as other RNs, LPNs. and non-licensed personnel. The nurse in charge must be able to effectively assess the skills and competencies of each team member. He or she must communicate in very clear terms what each member of the team must do. The RN will take responsibility for the outcome of the task.

Organization of Workload and Time Management

For an RN, organization and time management are non-negotiable. This is because the management of clients in a healthcare setting is usually time-bound. Triaging is a very important skill that every RN must master. For some clients, it is the difference between life and death.

Frameworks that can be used to prioritize include the following:

- CAB of resuscitation—cardiovascular or circulatory system, airway, and breathing. This is useful for deciding where to start when a practitioner is attending to a patient with cardiac arrest. However, it is important to note that the recent update has changed the sequence to CAB, meaning chest compressions to address cardiovascular or circulatory issues come first, followed by airway, and then breathing.
- Maslow's hierarchy of needs shows that the first thing to attend to is the patient's physiological needs, then safety, security, self-esteem, and self-actualization.
- Agency policies as dictated by the healthcare facility. Different healthcare institutions might come up with their own specific protocols for prioritizing patients. When this is done, the nurse must follow what has been stated and look for how this can be improved upon.
- Care should be prioritized so that all clients receive their medication promptly.

In addition, a nurse should be able to clarify whether an assignment is necessary. A nurse should also plan work systematically and make room for changes in the status or condition of clients and priorities.

All unnecessary interruptions should be avoided, and a nurse should learn how to decline tasks from other staff members when there are higher priority needs to be addressed. Without effective organizational skills, nurses burn out quickly or spend much time and energy on less important tasks.

Case Management

Case management in nursing involves developing, implementing, and evaluating healthcare plans for patients. But beyond this, it is an effective way to deliver nursing care. It typically involves managing and coordinating care, identifying and effectively utilizing resources, planning referrals, and connecting clients to services based on need.

Advocating for Cost-Effective Care

As case managers, nurses ensure that client care is high quality, cost-effective, and timely. It is the nurse's duty to explore all options with other healthcare team members to ensure that the patient is getting the most affordable care without a dip in quality.

There are two types of healthcare reimbursement: prospective and retrospective.

In the retrospective reimbursement system, healthcare facilities received payments for the care they rendered based on the actual costs that were incurred, and insurance companies were reimbursed for their services based on those costs. However, this was not sustainable as healthcare costs continue to rise globally.

The prospective reimbursement system came about to cut the excesses of retrospective reimbursement. Under this system, healthcare facilities are reimbursed a specific amount determined by the client's diagnosis. This has made more healthcare facilities conscious of how much is spent and makes them seek more efficient ways to cut costs and reduce the length of patient stays and resources used. Cost-effectiveness has become a priority for most healthcare organizations. Therefore, a nurse must understand it and utilize the fewest resources to produce the best results as much as possible.

Initiate, Update, and Evaluate the Plan of Care

Nurses are responsible for planning, updating, and evaluating healthcare plans for clients. The plan developed for each patient must be individualized based on the patient's condition and needs. The plan must take several factors about the client into consideration, such as the diagnosis, the patient's ability to take care of themselves, the currently prescribed treatment, actual and potential problems, and more. The plan must always remain up-to-date based on the current needs of the client.

As case managers, nurses ensure that all plans are carried out. This also includes the services performed by multidisciplinary team members who are not part of the nursing care team.

Nurses ensure that every patient is treated at the right level of care. They also educate clients and their families as needed, giving the reasons, the modalities, and the outcomes they are trying to achieve or prevent. If the goal is a discharge from the healthcare facility, the nurse ensures that clients and their families have enough information on what to do and what is expected at home or in the community.

The models that are used in case management include the following:

- The ProACT model: ProACT stands for the Professionally Advanced Care Team. The Robert Wood Johnson Foundation sponsored initiatives that are related to improving healthcare, but the specific ProACT model of case management is not directly attributed to the Robert Wood Johnson University Hospital.
- Collaborative practice.
- Case manager model.
- Triad model of case management.

Client Rights

Clients have rights and responsibilities that healthcare personnel must acknowledge to guide their practice.

Some client rights fall under the Self-Determination Act, which gives the patient the right to accept or reject care. Other rights include the following:

HIPAA

The Health Insurance Portability and Accountability Act (HIPAA) protects the personal information of clients, such as name, date of birth, social security number, and information on diagnosis and treatment. This act ensures that those who have access to the information are involved in the management or care of the patient.

Patient's Bill of Rights

The United States introduced the concept of a Patient's Bill of Rights in the 1970s. Here are some of the key areas that every nurse should be aware of:

1. Client information: Every client has the right to accurate and easy-to-understand information about the plan for their healthcare. It is important that clients know what is going on at every point in their care. If there is a communication barrier, such as a language difference, an interpreter should be provided to ensure patients clearly understand what is being done.

2. Choice of healthcare provider and healthcare plan: Every client has a right to choose the healthcare provider they want. They also have the right to choose the type of healthcare plan they prefer.

3. Access to emergency services: Every patient has the right to emergency screening and stabilization whenever they have an acute or severe condition. Patients have a right to these emergency services whenever and wherever they are needed, without authorization or financial penalties.

4. Making treatment decisions (informed consent): Patients have the right to know all available treatment options and decide which they prefer. They also have a right to select who can make decisions for them when they are not able to do so themselves. Patients should be clearly informed about their condition and the proposed treatment, which includes the benefits, risks, side effects, recovery, and any other information about the procedure.

5. Confidentiality: Patients have a right to speak privately to their healthcare providers and have their information treated confidentially. They have the right to look through their medical records and request an amendment of any inaccurate information.

6. Complaints and appeals: Patients have the right to a swift, fair review of any complaints they have against healthcare personnel or the facility.

7. Respect: Every client has a right to be treated with respect by healthcare professionals. They also have a right to be treated and attended to without discrimination from any healthcare worker.

Client Responsibilities

Client responsibilities include treating healthcare workers with respect, paying medical bills and other financial obligations as soon as possible, and reporting unexpected changes in their condition to the healthcare professional. They must also provide accurate information about their health, follow rules and regulations given upon admission, and be responsible for their own behavior.

A nurse must ensure that clients understand their rights and that the healthcare professionals also understand them.

Collaboration with a Multidisciplinary Team

Collaboration refers to the interdisciplinary interaction and cooperation between various sectors of healthcare. Nurses work with doctors, pharmacists, physical therapists, psychologists, social workers, nutritionists, and other healthcare professionals to achieve optimum client care and outcomes. To do this, there is a need to first take the following actions:

Identify the Need for Interdisciplinary Conferences

Interdisciplinary or multidisciplinary conferences involve interacting with other healthcare professionals involved in managing clients.

These meetings usually involve a lot of planning and the selection of an agenda, a date, a venue, and a fixed time. At these meetings, nurses can serve as patient advocates, raising issues that are pertinent to client care.

They can also resolve potential conflicts and areas of misunderstanding with other professionals. Interdisciplinary conferences are necessary for the holistic management of patients. They provide the opportunity to not only contribute to client care but also learn and observe from the perspective of other healthcare professionals. The goal is usually geared toward improving the delivery of client care.

In participating in interdisciplinary conferences, nurses should freely express their thoughts in a respectful manner while also listening to the points raised by other healthcare professionals.

Identify Significant Information to Report to Other Disciplines

In collaboration, there must be effective and timely communication between disciplines. Interdisciplinary client care will only thrive when there is smooth communication between healthcare professionals.

Nurses are on the front lines and will usually detect changes in patient conditions before other healthcare professionals. Hence, they must be able to communicate such observations promptly and clearly.

Nurses must know the signs to look out for in a patient's condition, whether it is in vital signs or reactions to prescribed drugs. They must then channel this information to the appropriate healthcare personnel for immediate action.

Review the Plan of Care to Ensure Continuity Across Disciplines

Nurses function as collaborators and managers of client care. Therefore, they are responsible for a continuous review of clients' care plans. Their review is to ensure that all healthcare professionals are doing what they should. If anyone defaults or deviates from the plan of care, then the nurse should point it out so that it can be corrected. It is important to note that this review must be continuous and up-to-date as the client's plan of care is being updated.

Collaborate with Multidisciplinary Team Members When Providing Client Care

Nurses collaborate with other members of the healthcare team to deliver quality healthcare. It is important that nurses maintain a high level of professionalism, good interpersonal and communication skills, and sound judgment when interacting with other healthcare professionals.

Some other team members and their roles include the following:

- **RNs**: Licensed healthcare personnel who are trained to deliver nursing care in several healthcare settings and who can manage both stable and unstable patients in structured or unstructured environments. They are also trained to coordinate other nursing team members, such as nursing assistants and LPNs.
- **Nursing assistants/patient-care technicians*:*** These are non-licensed assistants who help nurses provide direct and indirect care under the direct supervision of the RN. They also help perform non-sterile procedures requiring little technical expertise, such as collecting specimens, documenting vital signs, and ensuring patient movement and exercises and other patient activities required for daily living.
- **Licensed practical nurses**: Also licensed healthcare professionals, LPNs provide a wide variety of nursing care services in many different healthcare settings. They can perform both sterile and non-sterile procedures, and they can work with patients who are relatively stable in structured settings. They usually work under the supervision of an RN.
- **Nursing supervisors:** Nursing supervisors are responsible for patient supervision and receiving reports from several nurses under their supervision. They then pass these reports to the nursing director.

Additional professionals include medical doctors, doctors of chiropractic medicine, dieticians, physical therapists, occupational therapists, psychologists and social workers.

Serve as a Resource to Other Staff

Nurses can increase their effectiveness in collaborating with others by educating other members of the team. They can provide information about their areas of expertise and additional resources that will help other healthcare team members understand their roles and how to fit better into the healthcare team.

Medical doctors are licensed healthcare professionals who can provide primary care. They can also perform specialized roles, such as gynecology, cardiology, surgery, and more.

Physical therapists are licensed healthcare personnel who provide medical interventions concerned with a patient's functional abilities. They consider factors, such as strength, gait, and mobility, and use tools, such as walkers and exercise routines, to achieve their outcomes. They can practice in all healthcare settings, which includes the home setting.

Occupational therapists are closely related to physical therapists, but they focus more on interventions that help restore the client to the best possible level of independence. They are concerned with functions that contribute to daily living, such as eating, bathing, wearing socks, and getting dressed. Occupational therapists can work in all healthcare settings, which includes the home.

Social workers ensure that the client is appropriately moved in the continuum of care and there is no deficit after the patient is discharged. They counsel patients and can also provide psychological support. They are essential in cases of child abuse, neglect, or malpractice and can provide a much-needed link and support for victims.

Concepts of Management

Management is the process of hitting set targets by strategizing, organizing, and utilizing the efforts, talents, and resources available. Nurses have a set target to deliver and promote high-quality care to their patients. It is their responsibility as managers to ensure that they use whatever resources are available—both human and material—to achieve this. For managerial success, nurses must do the following:

Identify the Roles and Responsibilities of Healthcare Team Members

As discussed in other sections, healthcare personnel have different roles and responsibilities. It is the duty of the nurse to understand who plays what role and who handles what responsibilities. This way, when clients have needs, the nurse knows exactly who to call to provide the service.

If there is a need and the wrong person is called, it leads to wasted time and delays in delivering care. It also affects the schedule of the person who was mistakenly called.

Therefore, nurses should take understanding the roles and responsibilities of healthcare personnel very seriously.

Plan Overall Strategies to Address Client Problems

One important role of managers is to strategize. Client needs are important and can be overwhelming if there is no plan to attend to them. Therefore, nurses must come up with effective strategies to manage different client needs. These strategies must take into consideration the urgency of the task, as well as the personnel carrying it out.

Some of these strategies include the following:

- **Delegation and supervision:** As noted earlier, tasks should be delegated to personnel based on their skill level and competence.
- **The nursing process:** This includes planning, assessing, implementing, and evaluating, which should all be carried out efficiently.
- **Collaboration:** Nurses do not have the training required to attend to all client problems. Therefore, it is important to always reach out to other healthcare team members when a need arises that is peculiar to their specialty.
- **Educating clients and staff:** Nurses occupy a pivotal role, sometimes serving as the only link between clients and other staff. This places them in an advantageous position to educate both parties. Clients might need to be educated about their condition, the prognosis, the risks, expected interventions with their benefits and side effects, and more. The staff might need to be educated about the clients' rights and responsibilities and their own responsibilities toward the clients. They might also need to be educated on the patient's needs, how to solve them, and how to monitor for any change in their conditions. Client engagement is vital to obtain full cooperation. Patients tend to respond better when the healthcare team is more open and understanding.

Act as a Liaison between Clients and Others

Advocacy has been mentioned as one of the key elements of the nursing profession. Nurses serve as advocates for the client's family members, other members of the healthcare team, the management of the hospital, and even insurance companies. Their role as advocates is important to the managerial position they occupy.

Manage Conflict among Clients and Healthcare Staff

Conflicts or disagreements are a normal part of human interaction. They happen everywhere, and the healthcare setting is not exempt. Therefore, nurses must be skilled in managing conflicts among clients and healthcare staff.

Some of the most common causes of conflict in healthcare settings are the following:

- Disrespect.
- Overworking.
- Unfair distribution of roles or duties.
- Ill health.
- Patient loss.
- Negligence.
- Limited resources.
- Poor remuneration.
- Poor communication skills.
- Different personality types.

To resolve conflict, a nurse must understand the stages of conflict and conflict resolution, which include the following:

1. **Frustration:** The individuals involved in the conflict feel like their needs are being sidelined. It might be a need for respect, consideration of working hours, a bonus or raise, or a client feeling neglected.
2. **Conceptualization:** Those affected by the conflict begin to understand what is happening and why it happened. They begin to provide logical or illogical reasons that they believe caused the conflict.
3. **Action:** The individuals respond and act on the frustrations and conclusions that they have come to. At this point, the actions taken differ. For some, it

might be lashing out in anger or physical assault. Others might just withdraw.

4. **Resolution:** At this stage, all the people involved are able to come to an amicable solution.

Lewin's three types of conflict are based on approach and avoidance concepts.

A. **Avoidance-Avoidance conflict**: The individuals involved are not open to any of the alternatives that can lead to a resolution of the conflict. This might be because the alternatives are not appealing to either of the parties involved in the conflict.
B. **Approach-Approach conflict:** The individuals or parties involved have more than one alternative that can resolve the conflict. This is the direct opposite of the avoidance-avoidance conflict.
C. **Approach-Avoidance conflict:** The choices or alternatives that can resolve the conflict are not completely satisfactory to both parties. So, the choices have some positive aspects but also have some negative aspects.
D. **Double Approach-Avoidance conflict:** The involved individuals must choose one alternative due to its positive aspects but also accept the negative aspects while giving up other alternatives.

Healthy ways of resolving conflict include the following:

- **Collaboration and communication:** Conflicts will be easily settled when people in a healthcare setting are open to cooperating and working with each other. An environment of cooperation leads to better opportunities to air grievances and differences, and it fosters better relationships among members of the team.
- **Negotiation/Compromise:** Both parties must make a move to meet in the middle. This emphasizes focusing on common goals and interests, which in this setting should be the delivery of quality care rather than focusing on personal interests and desires. It also allows individuals to explore alternatives and offer solutions to a particular problem.
- **Mediation:** This requires an impartial third party to speak individually with those involved in the conflict before bringing them together to arrive at a

mutually beneficial conclusion. Many times, RNs might be required to play the role of mediators when there are conflicts.

The following are examples of ineffective or unhealthy methods of conflict resolution:

- **Avoidance:** Prolonged withdrawal and avoidance of the entire situation do not foster unity among the team members, nor do they lead to needs being met.
- **Competition:** Competition is very unhealthy for the healthcare team when it stems from conflict. It can put patient care at risk and reduce the quality of care.
- **Accommodating others without addressing issues:** While it is good to be accommodating and considerate, issues that are important to the individual should be resolved. If an individual continually neglects their unaddressed needs, their performance may suffer. Over time, this can result in resentment and other adverse reactions.

RNs must recognize patterns of conflict. If necessary, they should step in immediately to mediate the situation and prevent a deterioration of the relationship and ultimately the quality of care.

Evaluate Management Outcomes

As a manager, the goal is to always get more efficient with the use of resources. Therefore, evaluation and measurement must always be ongoing, and outcomes and results should always be measured. Were the set objectives met? Has the quality of care improved? Are the patients happy about a specific metric of care?

Confidentiality/Information Security

HIPAA protects the privacy and security of individuals' health information in the United States. It also gives patients rights over their health information, including the right to obtain a copy of their information and determine who can see it.

But this rule also balances the confidentiality of patient information with necessary disclosure for the provision of quality healthcare, for insurance, or for reimbursement.

Maintaining Client Confidentiality and Privacy

HIPAA provides legal protection for patients' medical records and limits the sharing of information by any means to those who need to know. The "need to know" population comprises those who need the medical information to render direct or indirect patient care and those the patient has documented in writing. Direct patient care refers to those who directly provide care to the patient, such as nurses, physical therapists, doctors, and others. Indirect care covers those who do not directly provide a form of care but still have a role to play in patient care, such as insurance providers, directors of nursing, and more.

Another aspect of maintaining client privacy is the privacy given to them during visits and in conversations with their families or guests.

In addition to HIPAA, healthcare facilities and institutions usually have their own regulations that help protect client privacy. Nurses should always maintain these regulations. Failure to do so can make a nurse liable for legal actions.

Assess Staff Member and Client Understanding of Confidentiality Requirements

One of the most effective ways to assess staff members' understanding of confidentiality requirements is by observation. As they carry out their daily routines, they observe the way they discuss patients and the way they use online medical records. Do they log out after finishing their task? Are they casual about opening client information anywhere? Do they talk about their patients online or post images of their patients on social media?

You can also assess clients' understanding of their rights regarding confidentiality by observing them. A client who asks for information about another client's case may not fully understand the principles of confidentiality in healthcare.

Intervene Appropriately When Staff Members Have Breached Confidentiality

A nurse is an advocate for the rights of the patient, and when any of these rights are breached, a nurse must be able to advocate for correction immediately.

Continuity of Care

Continuity of care refers to the seamless movement of a patient from one section to another in the same healthcare facility or from one healthcare facility to another. This continuity of care can be from a higher to a lower level of intensity of care or vice versa. It can be from a primary to a secondary or tertiary healthcare facility. The patient can also be discharged from the healthcare facility.

All these constitute transitions, which are referred to as continuity of care. At every level, care must be ongoing. The only difference is the type and intensity of care.

To ensure that this process is seamless, nurses have a major role to play in organization, communication, and collaboration.

Provide and Receive a Handoff of Care Report on Assigned Clients

It is essential to ensure a seamless transfer of patients at the end of shifts. The smooth handover of patient information is one of the basic elements of nursing care. This is because patient care is severely affected when a transfer is not seamless. It can affect medication plans, timing, and the overall quality of care. Hence, nurses must take this aspect of care seriously and go over every detail during the handover.

At the very minimum, reports should include the names of patients, the attending doctor's name, the admission date, and the diagnosis made. They should also include the completed and uncompleted tasks, care priorities, critical information about the health status of the patient, how responsive the patient has been to treatment, fluid input/output, observed unusual incidents, any special interventions, blood transfusion and if there was an adverse reaction, consults/referrals, and any alteration in the care plan or doctor's orders.

Highlighting all these might be cumbersome and difficult to remember during a handover. So, bodies, such as the Joint Commission on the Accreditation of

Healthcare Organizations, have come up with standardized handoff reports. They include the following:

- SBAR (situation, background, assessment, recommendations).
- ISBAR (introduction, situation, background, assessment, recommendation).
- BATON (background, actions, timing, ownership, next).
- IPASS (introduction, patient, assessment, situation, safety concerns).
- The five P's (patient, plan, purpose, problems, precautions).

All these provide a way of reporting essential information that must be passed on to the next nurse.

Use Documents to Record and Communicate Client Information

Documenting is pivotal to client care. In fact, some healthcare workers claim what is not documented is not done. A nurse must have a strong culture of documenting things. This is very important in the continuum of care. It provides a basis for assessment since what has been done and what is left to be done is clearly stated.

Different healthcare facilities have documents that they use as admission forms, vitals charts, fluid input and output forms, referral forms, discharge forms, and more.

It is the nurse's responsibility to understand the guidelines for each form.

Use Approved Terminology When Documenting Care

Another critical area to pay attention to is the terminology used in documentation. Sometimes, what is written is the only record available for healthcare. Therefore, great care must be taken to determine how something is written.

Healthcare facilities must have a list of permitted abbreviations and what they stand for to avoid misunderstandings and miscommunications. There should also be a list of prohibited abbreviations so that these are not used during documentation.

Perform Procedures Necessary to Safely Admit, Transfer, and/or Discharge a Client

Continuity of care basically involves admission, transfer, discharge, and referral of patients.

Admission refers to the initial client contact that results in a person entering the ward or healthcare facility. A transfer involves moving a patient from one section of the same healthcare facility to another. A discharge is a termination of care and services rendered on admission into healthcare. However, other services may continue. For instance, a patient might be discharged from the ward of a healthcare facility to the clinic of the same facility for regular check-ups or monitoring. A patient might also be discharged to another facility for follow-up.

Admission into a facility or ward will usually require that the client be thoroughly assessed, which includes the reasons for admission or transfer to another receiving section of the facility. It should involve detailed notes or reports from the transferring section or facility.

The nurse should educate the patient on the regulations of the healthcare section or facility, which includes the visiting hours, number of guests allowed, rules about privacy and confidentiality, use of restrooms, and more.

On discharge, there should be effective communication between the discharging section or facility and the receiving section or facility. There should be adequate documentation about the status of the patient on admission and then the status on delivery, noting the important changes that necessitated a discharge.

Other necessary documents from healthcare personnel should also be reviewed.

Follow-Up on Unresolved Issues regarding Client Care

Laboratory results and scans should all be followed up so that results are not missed. Nurses should always take follow-up seriously, and even if they are not able to resolve issues in their shift, they can communicate to the next nurse on shift or escalate the matter to higher authorities to be addressed.

Establishing Priorities

Establishing priorities is a skill every nurse must master.

Apply Knowledge of Pathophysiology When Establishing Priorities for Interventions with Multiple Clients

When handling multiple clients, the importance of evidence-based care cannot be overemphasized. The nurse should be familiar with disease and injury patterns and changes.

The knowledge of pathophysiology should guide the delivery of care. A nurse should understand changes that can occur, whether negative or positive, and when they are most likely to occur. These changes are either physiological or psychological, and they determine how health interventions will be carried out.

For instance, in attending to different clients with complaints in an emergency room, the nurse should bear in mind that patients who present with breathing difficulties should be attended to before people with minor cuts or bruises. And a patient who is on the verge of entering into shock will need swift attention compared to a patient who has the flu.

Checking for abnormal pulse rates, increased blood pressure, respiratory problems, or other diagnostic test values is also important.

In general, when a patient presents with certain complaints, knowledge of disease trends will aid in swift assessment, diagnosis, and planning of the client's care as necessary.

Prioritize the Delivery of Client Care Based on Acuity

When delivering quality care to a patient, acuity is vital for determining what comes first. Clients should be managed after identifying and differentiating biological needs from social needs.

For instance, in the admission of three clients into the ward, Client A is a postoperative patient with arrhythmia and uncontrolled pain, Client B is a new patient transferred to the ward from the outpatient clinic with stable vital signs, and Client C is a patient with a chest tube and on blood transfusion.

Prioritizing is based on the right knowledge, direct observation, vital assessment ratings, and tools within the healthcare practice.

Acuity helps in the critical thinking process and helps identify severe conditions that should take precedence in nursing interventions.

Evaluate the Plan of Care for Multiple Clients and Revise the Plan of Care as Needed

Evaluation is significant in nursing interventions. It finalizes the basis for acuity in client care. This first includes a thorough review of all the plans of care and treatment before the nurse can determine if new care plans are to be implemented.

Although evaluation is done at the end of the nursing process, it must not be overlooked because it implies whether an intervention was successful. Also, to perform proper evaluation, documentation must have taken place consistently throughout the patient's stay in the health facility.

In assessing and diagnosing multiple clients, which will eventually lead to continuity of care, it is important to analyze if all decisions made by the nurse in prioritizing care helped in the recovery.

Ethical Practice

Recognize and Report Ethical Dilemmas

Ethical dilemmas cannot be avoided in nursing practice. However, they can be duly recognized and reported while classifying each into the appropriate categories. Many of these issues are centered on protecting the rights of a patient, planning for palliative care, maintaining confidentiality and privacy, and involving clients in decision-making.

For instance, a patient in severe pain due to a femoral fracture and who has had an ORIF (open reduction and internal fixation) procedure is likely to request opioids or narcotics. This could pose a serious challenge to the nurse's profession and adherence to ethical standards, even while trying to serve the client's best interests.

Therefore, the nurse should be ready to report the situation to a superior to advocate for the patient's needs.

Also, in end-of-life scenarios, the nurse should discuss the prognosis of the illness before a decision is made in the interest of the patient. Here, detailed evidence of full disclosure should be documented.

Another example is the case study of a parent who refuses immunization for her child. No matter how attached the nurse is to the situation, after proper health education has been given to a parent who still refuses the vaccine, it is essential to report the entire process. This is done by documenting the education provided as well as a valid declaration of refusal despite all potential risks stated.

Inform Client and Staff Members of Ethical Issues Affecting Client Care

There should be an avenue to convey the right information about a health issue to a client or colleagues to ensure proper care planning, review, and continuity of care.

Practice in a Manner Consistent with the Nurses' Code of Ethics

The nurses' code of ethics provides guidance on behavior that is considered ethically and professionally appropriate for nurses. Therefore, the decision to elevate the standard of the profession while seeking to promote healthcare is vital.

The purpose of the code of ethics is to provide a framework for decision-making.

Various countries have nursing codes of ethics, such as the American Nursing Association (ANA), the Royal College of Nursing (RCN), and the International Council of Nurses (ICN), with a worldwide representation of professional nurse associations.

The fundamental responsibility of the nurse is to prevent illness, promote health, restore health, and alleviate suffering. Clients in need of nursing care should receive it without bias and with respect for life, human rights, and dignity.

This care should be given while also maintaining a cooperative relationship with colleagues in the profession and other medical practitioners in the field.

Evaluate Outcomes of Interventions to Promote Ethical Practice

The code of ethics is revised from time to time to include any developments or updates that take place. This includes changes in technology, the community, expansion of nursing practice into advanced practice roles, research, education, health policy, and administration.

Information Technology

Receive, Verify, and Implement Healthcare Provider Orders

One of the main obligations of the nurse to the client is to ensure that healthcare orders are accurately received and reported.

Nurses receive orders through diverse methods or channels. This could be through document format, electronic format, or other means.

It is vital that when these orders are received, the nurse checks for errors in the patient's age, allergies, diagnosis, medications, and routes of administration and verifies the right date of admission.

After receiving orders, the nurse is expected to verify them by asking for confirmation or clarity from healthcare providers. Inputting the information should be done with continuity of care in mind. Only then can the implementation of the orders take place.

Apply Knowledge of Facility Regulations When Accessing Client Records

All information about a client should be handled in line with the facility guidelines, even while handing it over to other colleagues or medical practitioners.

There should be no discussions with individuals who are not directly involved in clients' care.

Thus, personal privacy, which includes privacy during visits and during conversations, as well as securing electronic records with passwords, is highly recommended.

Access Data for Clients Through Online Databases and Journals

Obtaining information about clients' care through online databases helps provide a valid basis for the treatment and management of illnesses.

The nurse reviews a patient with the aid of a database to gain insight into better professional care, diagnostic procedures, clinical reports, and medication use.

Also, online databases and journals contain information and resources that are derived from evidence-based activities. Through this, the nurse gains access to scientific data by combining the best knowledge available from evidence, clinical experiences, and the patients' values.

Enter Computer Documentation Accurately, Completely, and Promptly

Computer documentation must be clear and precise. The nurse is expected to enter all vital information about a patient in an organized format from the time of admission until discharge.

This documentation is necessary to identify nursing interventions that have been provided to patients and to show patient progress during hospitalization. Other changes in patterns of care or administration should be documented as well.

Utilize Resources to Promote Quality Client Care (Evidence-Based Research, Information Technology, Policies, and Procedures)

Utilizing resources to improve healthcare, identify inefficiency, and promote performance assessment is vital.

Nurses use strategies and tools, such as electronic records and organizational procedures, that will help improve the quality of care rendered.

These resources help measure progress and evaluate the validity and reliability of the measures and sources of data received.

Legal Rights and Responsibilities

Nursing care comes with legal responsibilities.

Identify Legal Issues Affecting the Clients

Legal issues that affect clients are centered on the rights of a patient to be protected by the nurse and informed about any procedure to be carried out. For instance, in the case of a client who has refused treatment or demands discharge against medical advice, proper education, as well as documentation of evidence, are key. A nurse is expected to act in the best interest of the patient, per the principle of beneficence.

Identify and Manage Client Valuables According to Facility/Agency Policy

Upon discharge or termination of care, client valuables will be returned and must not be misplaced or mixed up. All items kept should be documented, with adequate descriptions and signatures of both parties involved.

Recognize Limitations of Self and Others and Utilize Resources

The legal system requires nurses to utilize resources provided to care for clients and not accept roles that do not fulfill nursing responsibilities.

For example, a client admitted into the hospital has a three-month-old baby. The client's husband pleads for the nurse to help care for the baby.

In this situation, the nurse can politely decline and refer the husband to a pediatric clinic. Legally, since the baby was not admitted along with the mother, the nurse cannot provide it with care.

The nurse should document that education about the client's baby's health was given and the baby was referred to the pediatric unit for further care.

Review Facility Policy and Legal Considerations before Agreeing to Serve as an Interpreter for the Staff or Primary Healthcare Provider

Clients who don't speak English may ask for translators or interpreters.

Nurses must understand all laws and regulations pertaining to interpreting. Although many states mandate provisions for sign language interpretation for the deaf, Braille is a system of raised dots that is read with the fingers and is specifically for people with visual impairments.

For federally funded facilities, clients have the right to an interpreter and should not be refused one. Documentation that the client understood all information is important to have and should include the date, time, name, and signature.

Educate Clients and Staff on Legal Issues

Professional bodies on ethical standards usually outline policies designed to prevent legal issues. The nursing officer is responsible for educating clients on the consequences of refusing care either for themselves or for family members, which must be reported and documented.

Likewise, all policies undergo legal reviews to set guidelines for nursing staff and other medical practitioners. This helps identify what is expected of caregivers and provides education on legal issues that could affect which services are or are not offered.

Report Client Conditions as Required by Law

The condition of a client on admission must be recorded in the client's chart. Incidents, such as abuse, gunshot wounds, road accidents, burns, harmful diseases, or cases of food poisoning, must be reported to the proper authorities. In violence- or abuse-related cases, an eyewitness may be able to provide information. Such information should be well documented for the authorities who can then carry out a detailed investigation.

Failure to report rape or sexual assault, theft, and injury could expose a nurse to charges of negligence.

Provide Care within the Legal Scope of Practice

All care a nurse provides should be within the legal scope of practice and properly documented. Informed consent should be received, and the confidentiality of the patient should be respected.

Although nurses often conduct certain laboratory tests like urine tests and glucose level checks as a part of their routine duties, they must ensure that they are working within their designated scope of practice and facility guidelines.

Performance Improvement (Quality Improvement)

Performance improvement focuses on enhancing and improving the quality and outcomes of care and increasing the efficiency of patient care while reducing costs, risks, and liabilities. Some steps in performance improvement include the following:

- Identify the improvement opportunity.
- Convene a team to carry out the quality improvement.
- Collect and analyze data.
- Explore the process under study.
- Eliminate variances that can negatively affect patient care

Define Performance Improvement/Quality Assurance Activities

Some important terms in understanding performance improvement include the following:

- **The culture of safety:** Any healthcare organization must have an established culture of safety, which must run from the top echelon of the organization to the employees.
- **A blameless environment:** A blame-free environment is required for performance improvement. A blameless environment is one where problems and mistakes are seen as opportunities for improvement. In this type of environment, the focus is not on the individual who made a mistake but on the different ways to improve the processes and workflow and make it fail-proof.
- **Root-cause analysis:** Very closely related to a blame-free environment is the root-cause analysis, which focuses on the cause of the problem. It is a process utilized in performance improvement activities that focuses on the "why" rather than the "who." The root-cause analysis focuses on the points of risk and vulnerability that are likely to result in errors in the healthcare organization. Root-cause analysis can only be carried out in a blameless environment.

- **Sentinel events:** A sentinel event refers to an incident or accident that led to or could potentially cause harm to a client. Examples of such events include the suicide of a client, abduction of infants, falls, wrong procedures performed, and adverse drug reactions, among others.
- **Variance tracking:** This process pinpoints and examines deviations for performance improvement. There are two types of variances: specific and random. Random variances arise unexpectedly and are not tied to a particular process or system flaw, whereas specific variances consistently emerge when a particular segment of a process is faulty or susceptible to human error.

Performance and Quality Indicators

Quality indicators are divided into core and outcome measures.

Core indicators are standard measurements of quality and reflect client populations, incidence of specific diseases, and organization. Outcome indicators focus on the outcomes of care after a patient has received healthcare. They include MRSA infection rates, lengths of stay, the effectiveness of fall prevention, and morbidity rates.

Risk management concentrates on the reduction and elimination of dangers and healthcare hazards that can result in liability for the company. Examples of these are infant abduction, patient falls, and medication errors. These risks can be identified and eliminated using root-cause analysis.

Participate in Performance Improvement Projects and Quality Improvement Processes

RNs may participate in performance improvement group activities that stress the importance of dependability, commitment, flexibility, communication, and discipline.

Performance improvement activities can follow several models, some of which include the following:

- The PDCA cycle involves planning, doing, checking, and acting.

- The Six Sigma method concentrates on problem definition, measurement, analysis of data, and improvements to make and control.

All these methods have some common features:

- Problem definition.
- Relevant data collection.
- Analysis of collected data.
- Root-cause analysis.
- Generation of possible solutions or alternatives.
- Selection of a solution or alternative with the greatest feasibility and highest chance of success.
- Evaluation of the effectiveness of the implemented solution.

Report Client-Care Issues to the Appropriate Personnel

Whenever there is an issue surrounding client care, nurses must promptly report it to the supervising nurse or whoever oversees the healthcare facility.

Most healthcare facilities have a structure for reporting client issues that includes the following:

- Channels of verbal communication through which concerns are orally communicated.
- Formal documents for reporting client concerns.
- Names and departments in charge of receiving such concerns.

When nurses report patient-care problems accurately and promptly, they ensure proper evaluation to detect the root cause of problems and prevent their reoccurrence.

Utilize Research and Other References for Performance Improvement Actions

Performance improvement activities require some research to see what other healthcare facilities are doing and to stay updated with current practices. Some resources that a nurse can utilize for reference and research purposes include published articles, research studies, standards of care and practice, published evidence-based practices, and relevant law and ethical codes. A nurse should serve as a source of improvement resources for the healthcare institution.

Evaluate the Impact of Performance Improvement Measures on Client Care and Resource Use

The impact of performance improvement activities should be measured. There are several ways to do this, which include the following:

- Compare the data before and after the corrective action.
- Evaluate whether the resulting action plans were effective in terms of increasing client safety, efficiency, and prompt delivery of care or decreasing costs or the number of patients involved in accidents or adverse events.
- Determine if the action plans were effective in the elimination of waste and the efficient use of resources at the appropriate level of care.

Referrals

Assess the Need for Referrals and Obtain Necessary Orders

Referrals are contacts that a nurse or other healthcare team members initiate so that the client's needs can be appropriately met at the required level of care and in the right setting.

It is the nurse's responsibility to ascertain when a referral is necessary and provide all the needed documentation and orders to ensure the process is seamless.

Assessing the Client

The first step in the referral process is to assess the client's needs and if the nursing staff and other healthcare professionals can adequately meet those needs. If a referral is needed, there should also be a reason for it. This could be due to a client's current problem or a potential problem that a client could face based on the trajectory of their condition.

Obtaining Necessary Orders

Once a need for referral is recognized, the RN should contact the appropriate internal or external resource who can meet the client's need. External resources can be a physical therapist or even a clergy member who can offer help.

A nurse must be able to recognize the appropriate resources for common referral needs, examples of which include the following:

- Individuals who have anger issues might need anger management programs.
- Uninsured clients might require social workers.
- Self-help groups in the community can be suggested for those who battle addiction or other mental health conditions.
- Shelters and housing can be recommended for clients who might be victims of abuse.
- Elder day care can be suggested for older patients.

Safety and Infection Control

Maintaining a safe and effective care environment is incomplete without having proper safety and infection control measures in place. These measures ensure that clients, as well as healthcare personnel, are protected from potential health and environmental hazards.

Accident/Error/Injury Prevention

Preventive measures are very important for safety and infection control. From accidents to injuries and administrative errors, there are many unfavorable incidents nurses can prevent from either occurring or escalating when they follow the right procedures during healthcare administration.

Preventive measures are extensive, and they begin even before a patient is admitted. They include setting up the right environment for effective patient care, planning for emergencies, anticipating and working to eliminate errors, and ensuring patient-specific risk factors as soon as a patient is admitted.

Assess the Client for Allergies and Intervene as Needed

Patients may be allergic to certain materials. Common allergies include medication and food allergies, latex reactions, and other reactions to materials and substances in the air.

Before administering care, patients should be assessed for existing allergies. This ensures only the safest procedures, equipment, and materials are utilized for individual patient care.

Nurses must also be able to recognize early signs of allergic reactions and what triggers they may be associated with. Certain reactions, known as anaphylactic reactions, can be life-threatening. It is therefore important that nurses immediately recognize these reactions and take necessary precautions.

Common allergy symptoms include but are not limited to swelling, numbness, itching or tingling at the exposure point, breathing difficulties, rashes or bumps, hypotension, and tachycardia. Swelling, numbness, or tingling sensations around the lips, mouth, or tongue usually indicate serious allergic reactions.

Nurses must also be aware of the appropriate intervention for each allergic reaction. Once an allergy is detected, it must be properly attended to, and the trigger must be removed immediately. Every allergic reaction must be documented to inform future healthcare measures.

Assess the Client-Care Environment

The client-care environment is the physical and social setting in which nursing care is provided. Assessing the client-care environment involves considering factors, such as safety, comfort, privacy, and cultural sensitivity.

Safety is a priority, and nurses should ensure that healthcare environments are continually kept safe from threats and potential hazards. The environment must be regulated to minimize falls and other injuries. Materials and equipment used should be sterile or properly disinfected before reuse, and all allergens must be removed.

The environment should also be checked for factors that can trigger self-harm or aggression in patients.

The client-care environment must be assessed to ensure physical and emotional comfort. Bedding and other facilities provided should be comfortable for each patient's unique condition. Privacy must be maximized, and the care environment should support patient confidentiality.

Note that assessing the client-care environment is a process that needs to be done continuously—before patients are admitted, while they are in the facility, and after they've been discharged.

Determine Client and Staff-Member Knowledge of Safety Procedures

Both clients and healthcare workers should be assessed for their knowledge of the right safety procedures for each situation. This can be done by conducting surveys in the form of questionnaires, group discussions, and one-on-one interactions.

Staff members should be adequately trained to attend to patients with safety and infection control in mind. All staff members must be aware and updated on policies and procedures for ensuring safety and should be continuously trained to manage situations effectively.

On the other hand, clients should be properly guided on how to deal with their unique situations and avoid escalations. Educational materials can be developed in simple and accessible forms for patients, caregivers, family members, and friends.

Identify Factors That Influence Accident and Injury Prevention

Some situations serve as risk factors for accidents and injuries. These include factors, such as the patient's developmental stage, lifestyle, and mental health status. Children and the elderly are more prone to accidents and injuries than adults, while the mental health status of some patients can make them prone to self-inflicted injuries.

Nurses should remain aware of these factors and work to ensure they do not trigger patient accidents.

Identify Deficits That May Impede Client Safety

Hearing, sensing, and perception deficits must be identified and considered when administering care to patients. Patients with deficits might require care in special environments with close supervision to prevent accidents. Patients who use assistive equipment must be placed in ideal environments and properly monitored to ensure their assistive devices do not become potential risk factors.

Identify and Verify Orders for Treatments That May Contribute to Accident or Injury

Certain treatments and procedures aside from medication may contribute to accidents, injuries, and other negative health incidents in patients. Nurses can check this by monitoring the patient's conditions to identify treatments that might become risks and determine the best procedures for treatment.

Each patient's medical history should be reviewed for information, such as underlying health conditions, allergies, and other adverse reactions, that certain treatments can trigger. All new findings should be properly documented to guide future healthcare measures.

Identify and Facilitate the Correct Use of Infant and Child Car Seats

Car seat laws and requirements for infants and children can vary by state. However, many laws often require infants and toddlers to use car seats based on age, height, or weight criteria, but the specifics can vary by state. Nurses must stay aware of specific requirements in their states and should educate parents and guardians on the proper use of car seats and other safety measures for children.

Promote Staff Safety

The process of ensuring a safe and secure environment for healthcare is not complete without looking out for the safety of staff members. Without the right measures, staff members can become potential safety and infection threats to patients and their families and vice versa.

Here are a few things that can be done to promote staff safety:

Provide education and training: Providing education and training to staff members on safety procedures, which include emergency codes, infection control, and workplace violence prevention, is highly important not just for the safety of patients but also for the staff's own safety and well-being.

Provide personal protective equipment (PPE): Providing staff members with appropriate PPE, such as gloves, gowns, masks, and goggles, ensures maximum protection from infectious and other hazardous materials. Not only should these provisions be made available, but staff members should be trained on how to properly wear, remove, dispose of, or prepare PPE for reuse.

Create a safe and ideal work environment: All equipment should be properly maintained and in good working order. Hazards and obstacles should be removed, and adequate lighting should be provided in all areas of the healthcare facility.

Encourage staff communication: Staff members should be encouraged to communicate any safety concerns they may have, such as hazards in the work environment or concerns about patient behavior. There should be an open and supportive environment that makes staff members feel comfortable speaking up.

Provide Clients with Appropriate Methods to Signal Staff Members

Patients should be provided with the right methods to use to signal staff members and ensure they can communicate their needs and receive assistance when necessary.

Here are some key methods for signaling staff members:

- Call bells.
- Communication boards.
- Intercom systems.
- Bedside monitors.
- Personal emergency response systems (PERS).

Protect Clients from Injury

Patients have a high chance of injury in the healthcare environment. Therefore, it is important for nurses to watch out for these risk factors, provide options for mitigating them, and educate clients on how to request assistance or avoid falls and other kinds of injuries.

Appropriate care workers and other staff workers should be positioned in key locations, such as bathrooms and showers, and families and friends should be enlightened on important safety measures.

The healthcare environment should be designed to minimize risk factors for falls and injuries. This includes the provision of handrails in bathrooms and showers, guard rails on patients' beds, appropriate lighting, alarms so patients can alert healthcare workers in the event of a fall or any other type of injury, minimal room and floor clutter, the removal of hazardous substances, and ensuring that all equipment is in good working order.

Assistive devices should be recommended and provided for those who need them. Clients should be trained on how to install, uninstall, and properly use these devices. Lastly, medication should be administered safely and professionally. Nurses should check medication orders for accuracy, verify medication dosages, and monitor clients for potential side effects.

Review Necessary Modifications to Reduce Stress on Specific Muscle or Skeletal Groups with Clients

Due to extended periods of immobility, patients may begin to experience stress on specific muscle or skeletal groups. Nurses can help facilitate stress reduction in their clients and make them more comfortable by encouraging them to perform routine muscular and skeletal exercises, such as stretching and frequently changing positions.

Patients who are at risk for pressure ulcers and are unable to change their positions by themselves should be turned approximately every two hours. Such clients should also be assisted in performing stretching exercises so strength and mobility can be preserved.

Clients and their caregivers should be instructed which positions and bodily alignments are the best to maintain. These include the Sim's or semi-prone position, the prone position, the Fowler's position, the lateral position, and the dorsal recumbent position. They should also be taught how to use supports, such as pillows, wedges, and bolsters.

Implement Seizure Precautions for At-Risk Clients

Nurses should implement seizure precautions for patients who are at risk. These precautions include identifying and removing environmental triggers, removing dangerous materials patients can latch on to during seizures, lowering the patient's bed to the lowest setting or placing the mattress on the ground, using beds with padded side rails, and always having oxygen and suction equipment at the patient's bedside.

Intervention procedures during a seizure recommend that a patient should be put into a side-lying position to prevent aspiration. Oxygen should only be administered if there are signs of respiratory distress or hypoxia.

Make Appropriate Room Assignments for Cognitively Impaired Clients

Cognitively impaired clients should be admitted to rooms that allow for close monitoring. The rooms must be designed to prevent accidents and injuries and ensure easy access to treatment and medical observations.

Properly Identify Clients when Providing Care

It is important to properly identify clients when providing care to avoid errors, such as mismatched prescriptions, which can be life-threatening.

It is recommended to have at least two distinct identifiers aside from the room number of clients. Instead of room numbers, nurses should consider using patients' full names, complete dates of birth, and other unique identification measures.

Nurses should also be mindful of patients who are at higher risk of identification errors. These include patients who cannot communicate in English, cognitively impaired patients, and patients who have similar names as other registered patients.

Verify the Appropriateness and Accuracy of a Treatment Order

Nurses must never be in a hurry or careless about administering treatment. They should verify the appropriateness and accuracy of each treatment order, especially when they appear out of place or questionable. Nurses should reach out to the healthcare personnel who have prescribed such treatments or procedures for proper verification. To be successful at this, nurses must be aware of what medication and prescriptions are appropriate for each patient based on factors, such as age, stage of disease, and more.

Emergency Response Plan

The Joint Commission requires every healthcare facility to have an emergency response plan. This, in turn, demands every staff member understand and be properly drilled on how to handle emergency situations effectively.

Identify Nursing Roles in Disaster Planning

Nurses must be prepared to handle all kinds of emergencies, which include those inside medical facilities, such as fire, workplace violence, radiation contamination, building collapse, and utility failures. These are known as internal disasters. Nurses must also be prepared to handle external emergencies, such as disease outbreaks, fires, wars, natural disasters, and other mass casualty events.

The role of a nurse in the face of disaster and other emergencies may vary, but it will include attending to affected casualties and preventing the escalation of harm to patients and staff. To do this, nurses may be assigned to perform triage, administer treatment, track patient health, and discharge patients as soon as possible to provide room for more casualties.

In certain disasters, nurses will teach volunteers basic first aid and caregiving principles to ease the burden of professional medical staff members while ensuring they can focus on the most critical situations.

The primary role of a nurse in the face of disaster is to ensure patients are not just treated but also kept safe from further harm.

Determine Which Clients to Recommend for Discharge in a Disaster

During mass casualty events, it is common to have many patients awaiting treatment. Nurses should use critical thinking and their knowledge of triage to ensure all patients are attended to, even in such difficult situations.

Priorities should be set to determine patients who should be recommended for quick discharge or relocation, while the most critical patients should be attended to first.

Ambulatory clients who are medically stable and require little to no assistance can be considered for early discharge after they have been treated and given prescriptions as needed. Unstable patients are high priority and are therefore not candidates for discharge. Stable patients who still require medical care and assistance should also be considered for admission into the facility. In the event of a lack of space, however, they may be carefully relocated to other available facilities while being strictly monitored.

Use Clinical Decision-Making/Critical Thinking for an Emergency Response Plan

All RNs must be aware of how their decisions can impact the well-being of patients, whether positively or negatively. They must always deploy critical thinking and sound decision-making skills, especially in emergency situations.

Participate in Emergency Planning and Response

Nurses participate in emergency planning and help implement response plans in such emergencies. To make effective plans, nurses must stay aware of their roles in accordance with the policies applicable in their locality.

These policies inform nurses about how they can get involved in planning and preparing for emergencies. Nurses should engage in drills and practices that mimic common emergency situations within or outside the healthcare environment.

Nurses must stay up-to-date on the appropriate emergency protocols for each situation, which include evacuation procedures and communication systems. Communication is an important component of a successful emergency response plan. Each healthcare organization may have prescribed procedures for communication in different emergency situations. Nevertheless, nurses should be able to use intuition to discern and plan the most effective ways to communicate during emergencies to avoid further risks.

Many organizations utilize code names to communicate different emergency situations quickly and efficiently. These codes serve as a standardized method to alert staff and initiate appropriate responses. Here are a few examples:

- **Code Blue:** This code is commonly used to indicate a cardiac arrest or a medical emergency that requires immediate resuscitation.
- **Code Red:** This code is typically used to signify a fire or the presence of smoke within the facility and prompts immediate evacuation and fire response protocols.
- **Code Orange:** When there is a chemical spill or release of hazardous materials, Code Orange is often used to alert personnel and initiate appropriate containment and decontamination procedures.
- **Code Pink:** This code is commonly associated with infant abduction or the disappearance of a newborn and triggers a coordinated effort to locate and ensure the safety of the infant.
- **Code Gray**: Although some organizations may use Code Gray for severe weather conditions or preparedness measures for events like hurricanes and intense storms, others may use it to refer to situations like a combative person or potential violence. It's important to be aware of the specific definitions used by each individual institution.

Ergonomic Principles

Use Ergonomic Principles When Providing Care

Nurses should consider ergonomic principles and body mechanics when they provide care to clients and help them use assistive devices. All devices, facilities, and equipment should allow patients, their caregivers, and other healthcare workers to safely move from one point to another or move distinct body parts.

Ergonomic principles should be observed when nurses undertake the following tasks:

- Move patients from one point to the other on stretchers and wheelchairs.
- Help patients maintain a comfortable position to receive healthcare. This could be lying down, sitting down, or standing.
- Help patients on machines and operating tables.
- Choose the right assistive device for each patient's needs.
- Provide therapy to patients.

Note that ergonomic principles do not benefit patients alone. For example, the right application of procedures for moving patients from one point to another will also prevent injuries and strain on nurses and other healthcare workers.

Here are a few things nurses should note when handling patients and using common hospital equipment and facilities:

- Stretch or warm up before lifting a client or heavy objects.
- Review actions and what the best procedure for execution might be.
- Collaborate with other healthcare workers or caregivers. Explain the task and the desired results. Communicate with patients so they can physically and emotionally prepare themselves for the activity. In some situations, a patient may even be able to participate in the process, bending, shifting, and twisting when needed.
- Always face the person or object you are about to move or lift unless you are working in a group and your positioning at the time might not permit you to face the client.
- Keep key body parts, such as the spine, neck, back, and head aligned when lifting. Avoid twisting.

- When lifting, provide a secure base for supporting yourself by keeping your feet apart.
- Keep a secure grip on the object or client you will lift.
- Use your arm and leg muscles to lift, not your back.
- Use mechanical lifts and appropriate assistive devices when available.

Assess Clients' Ability to Balance and Transfer and Use an Assistive Device Prior to Planning Care

Before assistive devices, such as crutches, walkers, braces, and hearing and visual aids, are assigned to patients, they must be tested for client suitability and convenience. Factors, such as cognitive ability and muscular strength, could impact a person's ability to balance and use some devices.

Therefore, every assistive device assigned to a patient must meet individual needs, such as developmental stage, height, weight, and terrain. Each patient must also be properly instructed on how to use and manage their assistive devices.

Provide Instruction and Information to Clients about Body Positions That Eliminate the Potential for Repetitive Stress Injuries

Repetitive stress injuries occur due to repeated movement or overuse of certain muscles or muscle groups. They typically occur due to the postures patients maintain over time or due to placing weight or applying pressure on certain parts of the body over time. Repetitive stress injuries cause cramping, stiffness, and neurological discomfort and might lead to complications when not properly addressed.

Patients should be taught to maintain anatomically correct positions and should be made aware of their new limits or restrictions, if any.

Handling Hazardous and Infectious Materials

Hazardous materials include both non-biological and biological materials that pose some form of risk to human beings, animals, and other living things. They can be anything from harmful chemicals and radiation to soiled and used equipment, such as needles, that could become potential sources of infection.

RNs are instrumental in ensuring that these materials, in all their forms, do not pose any risk to clients.

Identify Biohazardous, Flammable, and Infectious Materials

The U.S. Occupational Safety and Health Administration (OSHA) requires that workers in healthcare environments have firsthand information about hazardous materials, what risks they may pose, and what actions to take in the case of exposure. Nurses and other healthcare workers must also be able to identify these hazardous materials and how to handle them.

Biohazardous materials are biological waste and items that have been contaminated with biological waste that can be harmful to humans. Used hospital bedding, tubes containing bodily fluids and excretions, and used needles are all examples of biohazardous waste.

Biohazardous, flammable, explosive, and infectious materials are regulated at national, state, and local levels. Healthcare facilities should comply with the policies available to their region for labeling, storing, disposing, and managing these wastes.

All hazardous materials should be properly labeled such that even lay personnel are able to identify the risks.

Follow Procedures for Handling Biohazardous and Hazardous Materials

Each biohazardous material comes with unique procedures for handling, transporting, disposing of, and disinfecting if applicable. Some waste needs to be destroyed as soon as it is used. Other waste can be disinfected before final disposal, while still other waste can be disposed of in containers and made ready for safe reuse. It is therefore important that nurses follow the right protocols and procedures for handling waste.

There are general principles for handling biohazardous waste that apply in all healthcare systems. The following are some of the most important principles:

- Rigorous handwashing after handling any biohazardous material.
- Proper allocation of trash cans in patient rooms and at strategic points in the healthcare facility for easy waste disposal.
- Proper disposal of materials, such as needles and latex gloves, designed for single use.
- Proper cleaning and disinfection of non-single-use materials, such as certain PPE, that come in contact with biological waste.
- Proper disposal of biohazardous material in accordance with stipulated national, state, and local laws.
- Proper procedures to ensure proper disposal of each kind of waste.
- Safe transportation and proper labeling of hazardous and flammable substances, such as oxygen tanks.
- Education for clients and their caregivers on handling and disposing of biohazardous waste, such as used bedding and bodily fluids.

Demonstrate Safe Handling Techniques to Staff and Clients

The RN may be obligated to demonstrate how to safely handle hazardous substances to other staff members in the healthcare environment, as well as to clients who are receiving healthcare. In such situations, the nurse assumes the role of an educator, assesses the learning needs of concerned parties, and demonstrates appropriate techniques for handling hazardous materials.

Ensure Safe Implementation of Internal Radiation Therapy

Long exposure to radiation poses dangerous health risks. Nurses work with radiation therapists and other professionals and follow safety guidelines to minimize exposure to radiation.

There are three major ways to ensure safety during radiation therapy: time, distance, and shielding. Nurses and technicians should ensure clients have minimal exposure to radiation by minimizing exposure time, ensuring safe distance, and using shielding.

It is also important to implement safe interaction of caregivers, family, friends, and other patients with clients currently being treated with radiation therapy.

Home Safety

Healthcare does not end at the healthcare facility. Nurses are vital in ensuring clients have appropriate instructions to ensure a safe transition to the home environment.

Assess the Need for Client Home Modifications

Nurses, alongside other healthcare staff, such as physical therapists, discharge planners, and counselors, work together to assess clients' homes, identify safety concerns, and offer solutions or modifications.

Factors, such as lighting, handrails, slip-proof floors, oxygen tanks, and emergency exits, are critical to improving the well-being of patients and helping them adjust their lifestyles to the new health conditions they may be managing.

Apply Knowledge of Client Pathophysiology to Home Safety Interventions

Certain diseases and disorders require unique provisions so clients can better manage these situations. Patients with cognitive disabilities might require close monitoring and may be prevented from exposure to materials that could potentially cause harm to them or others around them. Clients with perceptual deficits will also require special aids that will promote their safety, help them handle emergency situations, and help them interact with their environment more effectively.

Educate Clients on Safety Issues

Many clients are unaware of what potential risks their daily routines and lifestyles might impose on their health. Nurses must determine each client's level of knowledge about home safety needs and provide adequate education.

Clients may be presented with written instructions or other teaching aids that will serve as a resource they can always return to.

Encourage Clients to Use Protective Equipment When Using Devices That Can Cause Injury

Clients should be educated on the right protective equipment to use for each high-risk activity and should be strongly encouraged to always use this equipment. Protective equipment applicable for home use includes simple items, such as hand gloves and safety goggles. Clients should also be encouraged to properly dispose of sharps and other biohazardous wastes.

Evaluate Client-Care Environment for Fire and Environmental Hazards

Patient-care environments must be properly evaluated for fire and other environmental hazards. Such hazards must be eliminated when possible, while other needed healthcare materials must be correctly labeled to inform healthcare personnel of the risks. Lastly, fire safety equipment must always be available and within reach.

Reporting an Incident/Event/Irregular Occurrence/Violence

Nurses must always report irregular events, cases of violence, and other uncommon incidents, depending on the applicable protocol at their workplace. Usually, such reports must go to the supervising or charge nurse and the risk management department in the healthcare facility.

Providing these reports helps ensure issues are promptly addressed and can be prevented in the future. They also help with record-keeping and tracking trends.

Details that should be included in formal reports for incidents and other irregular occurrences include the following:

- The date, time, and place the event occurred.
- A brief background on what triggered the event, such as an object that a client tripped on, for example.

- The name of the individual affected by the event.
- The nature of injuries sustained.
- The names of the witnesses present.
- The care and treatment procedures that were used.
- The names of healthcare workers who were contacted to attend to the event.

Identify Needs/Situations Where Reporting of an Incident/Event/Irregular Occurrence Is Appropriate

All significant or concerning events should be recorded, even if they seem routine or minor. Here are some examples:

Practitioner variance: This is a consequence of activities or services of a healthcare provider. An example would be delayed attendance to a client until complications occur.

System or institutional variance: This is associated with an issue originating with the healthcare facility. A prime example is inadequate supplies or a shortage of staff members that results in substandard patient care.

Patient variance: This is associated with issues originating with the client. For example, unexplainable and sudden complications or an event that occurs because a client has not adhered to a treatment routine.

Acknowledge and Document Practice Errors and Near Misses

RNs, as well as other healthcare providers, must always remain responsible and own up to human errors in the workplace. These errors, when identified, should be properly documented with details on the exact nature of the error, the consequences that accompanied it, and the current state of those affected by the error.

Errors and near-misses remain underreported in healthcare facilities. This is due to various factors, such as fear of owning up and getting penalized, ignorance of the error itself, and ignorance of how to go about documenting such errors. Proper documentation can, however, help inform intervention procedures, which include how healthcare workers should be trained to reduce the frequency of such errors.

Evaluate Response to Error/Event/Occurrence

The RN must evaluate a client's response to an error or negative event as soon as it has been identified. At times, clients may be unable to provide information on the effects of such events because they are unconscious, unaware of their situation, or too indisposed to communicate.

The nurse should perform a thorough evaluation to identify the patient's current state while paying attention to priority needs first. The patient's state at the time of the event should be recorded, and progress should be tracked over time.

Report, Intervene, and/or Escalate Unsafe Practices of Healthcare Personnel

RNs are responsible for looking out for other healthcare workers and reporting out-of-place behaviors and unsafe practices that could pose threats to clients and other persons in the healthcare environment. Such unsafe practices include substance abuse, improper care, biases directed toward certain clients, degenerating health and mental state of a health worker, and so on.

Safe Use of Equipment

The condition of equipment used in the healthcare environment and how staff members can manage such equipment go a long way toward preventing hazards, client complications, and injuries to healthcare workers.

Inspect Equipment for Safety Hazards

The maintenance or equipment department usually conducts thorough inspections and evaluations of all equipment used by staff or clients. Nurses can ensure that these inspection procedures have been observed and should pay attention to instructions and operation procedures, which include preliminary checks that are necessary before using any equipment.

Nurses should particularly look out for frayed electrical cords, overloaded power outlets, loose or missing equipment parts, and other questionable conditions that could pose a threat.

Teach Clients About the Safe Use of Healthcare Equipment

Both clients and staff members should be properly trained to handle and manage whatever equipment they may be called to use. They should also learn how to identify potential threats and handle quick fixes if applicable, as well as what to do if complications arise.

Clients should be trained on how to safely handle equipment, particularly any they will use at home away from staff members' oversight. This equipment should be thoroughly checked before being provided to clients, and clients should be taught how to conduct routine checks. Depending on the nature of the equipment or device, patients may also be instructed to bring it in for inspection or replacement during their next health check.

Facilitate Appropriate and Safe Use of Equipment

RNs can help facilitate the appropriate and safe use of equipment by following these directives:

- Learn how each piece of equipment works.
- Ensure they do not operate any equipment unless they have been trained to handle it.
- Perform routine inspections on equipment before use and report malfunctions as soon as they are discovered.
- Do not use equipment or devices deemed faulty.
- Educate other staff members about how to handle equipment when they need to use it.
- Educate clients on how to properly manage equipment and assistive devices.

- Report equipment that is faulty or out of service so it can be labeled accordingly or removed to prevent another staff member from using it.

Security Plans

Security planning is an important aspect of healthcare. An excellent security plan ensures lives and property at the facility are secure.

Use Clinical Decision-Making/Critical Thinking in Situations Related to Security Planning

Once again, critical thinking and excellent decision-making skills are vital in security planning. The RN is a key participant in the planning, execution, and evaluation of security procedures and must be able to always offer working solutions.

In accordance with regulations and recommendations, healthcare facilities must create working security plans. Bodies responsible for providing security regulations include the JCAHO and the International Association for Healthcare Security and Safety. The Centers for Medicare and Medicaid oversee health coverage, quality standards, and other related matters.

Nurses must remain fully aware and updated about the security plans in their facility, which include codes for communicating situations and what to do in the event of a security threat.

Apply Principles of Triage and Evacuation Procedures and Protocols

In the event of a security threat, nurses must apply principles of triage to create a protocol that caters to the most critical clients first. These include immobile clients who may be unable to escape threats on their own or those who have been critically injured due to such threats. As explained in the principles of triage, medically unstable patients are to be attended to first, followed by stable patients who still require assistance, and lastly, ambulatory clients who do not require assistance.

Follow the Security Plan and Procedures

Security threats are a unique form of emergency, and nurses must always be prepared to combat them. Key ways to do this are periodic trainings; reviewing policies, procedures, and recommendations for different security situations; and participating in mock sessions to prepare for situations, such as access breaches, violence, and property or human theft.

Standard Precautions/Transmission-Based Precautions/Surgical Asepsis

Infection control is just as important as other safety measures. Because the healthcare environment is one where patients and healthcare providers interact with several potential infection risk factors at once, it is very important to ensure that infections are not transmitted from one patient to another, between healthcare personnel, or from patients to healthcare personnel and vice versa.

There are several procedures for infection control, such as maintaining a strict surgical asepsis routine, properly disposing of biohazardous waste, and following standard and transmission-based precautionary measures.

Understand Communicable Diseases and the Modes of Organism Transmission

Diseases are transmitted when an etiologic agent, that is, a pathogen capable of causing an infection, is transmitted from a current host or reservoir to a new or susceptible host. Disease-causing agents include bacteria, fungi, viruses, protozoa, and helminth parasites. These agents go through a chain of transmission from the reservoir to the portal of exit, to the mode of transmission to the portal of entry, and finally to the susceptible host. This is known as the chain of infection.

The portal of exit is the point through which the agent or pathogen leaves the reservoir, while the portal of entry is the point through which the agent enters a susceptible host. These portals can include body orifices or systems and activities, such as sneezing or vomiting.

When pathogens leave through the portal of exit of a reservoir, they may gain access to the portal of entry of a new host, such as another patient, a medical staff member, or family, friends, and well-wishers of patients.

The mode of transmission is the specific medium through which the infectious agent is transmitted from the reservoir to a new host. These are the modes of transmission of pathogens:

- Contact (direct and indirect).
- Airborne.
- Droplet.
- Vector-borne.

Assess Client-Care Area for Sources of Infection

RNs must continually monitor and assess the client-care area for potential sources of infection while providing healthcare to patients. Infection sources and risk factors for infections should be properly communicated and the right measures for preventing, testing for, or treating such infections should be taken immediately.

Because nurses and other staff members are important figures in transmitting healthcare-acquired infections, they must strictly follow preventive procedures, which include frequent handwashing and the use of PPE.

Apply Principles of Infection Prevention

There are several provisions for infection prevention and control to which nurses must strictly adhere at all times. These include the following:

Hand hygiene: Hand hygiene is the most effective procedure for preventing the spread of infection. Proper hand hygiene, such as washing with soap and water or using an alcohol-based hand rub, prevents thousands of infections from spreading in healthcare environments. Protective gloves are a part of additional precautions but do not replace the need for good hand hygiene. Nurses should note that, unlike medical equipment that can be sterilized, the hands and other parts of the skin cannot be sterilized. They can only be sanitized. Sterilization procedures, such as the use of bleach and other chemicals, are harmful to the skin and could cause irritation or more serious skin concerns.

Handwashing should be done in all the following situations:

- Before and after contact with a client.
- Before and after removing gloves.
- After touching equipment, instruments, and other treatment materials with bare hands.
- When hands have been soiled with bodily fluids, secretions, and chemicals.

Aseptic techniques: Aseptic techniques or medical asepsis are measures taken in addition to standard and transmission-based precautions to prevent the transfer of disease-causing organisms from one person or object to another. Aseptic techniques include barriers, patient and equipment preparation, environmental controls, and contact guidelines. They differ from sterile techniques, which are measures for neutralizing infectious microorganisms. Sterile techniques are usually applied during surgical procedures and invasive wound care.

Universal/Standard precautions: These are recognized infection control measures for preventing infection spread among clients, whether or not they've been diagnosed with any infection.

Transmission-Based precautions: These are preventive and infection control measures that are utilized to combat and inhibit the spread of specific infections. These precautionary procedures are informed based on the type of infection and its medium of transmission.

PPE: This is specialized equipment used to protect specific body areas from injury and exposure to infectious agents. Examples of PPEs are gloves, goggles, masks, respirators, aprons, face shields, and gowns. Nurses should observe basic principles for donning, removing, disposing of, and sterilizing personal PPE as appropriate. They should also wash their hands before and after using PPE.

Follow Correct Policies and Procedures When Reporting a Client with a Communicable Disease

Infectious diseases can spread very quickly and become a major threat to the whole community. Nurses should follow the regulations that apply to reporting and communicating diseases. Usually, reports about communicable diseases, epidemics, and other outbreaks are submitted to appropriate local or state health departments, which may then relay relevant information to the Centers for Disease Control and Prevention.

Educate Clients and Staff Regarding Infection Prevention Measures

RNs educate clients and staff members on infection prevention and control measures directly and indirectly. They assess the educational needs of these groups and plan educational activities to meet those needs. They also evaluate the impact and effectiveness of such educational sessions on infection prevention and control.

Nurses may educate clients on infection prevention measures based on their specific health needs, current healthcare routine, and life situation. They teach clients how to properly dispose of biohazardous waste and how to perform asepsis and other standard or treatment-based precautions.

Nurses are responsible for helping patients and their family members understand the importance of certain infection control and prevention measures, such as isolation and the need for family members to wear a gown or other PPE before accessing treatment wards.

Use Appropriate Precautions for Immunocompromised Clients

Immunocompromised clients are at a higher risk of contracting infection after exposure. Other factors, such as an immune-deficiency disease, age, medications, and certain therapeutic interventions, such as radiation and chemotherapy, increase this risk.

Immunocompromised clients are given special care and prevented from contact with infectious agents that might not pose a threat to non-compromised clients. Stringent infection control measures should be practiced for these clients. They may need to be isolated from other people until they have attained some level of recovery and immunity.

Use the Appropriate Technique to Set Up a Sterile Field/Maintain Asepsis

Nurses may assist or manage the setup of a sterile field during surgical asepsis. Here are the appropriate techniques and procedures to follow:

- Only sterile items should be placed on the sterile field.
- The nurse should never have the sterile field below the waist level or above the chest level.
- The nurse should not lean over or turn their back to the sterile field.
- Coughing or sneezing over the sterile field contaminates it.
- There should be a one-inch border of sterile space around the sterile field. It is within this space that sterile items are placed.
- Moisture or wetness contaminates the sterile field. It must always remain dry.
- Sterile liquids should be carefully poured into sterile containers on the sterile field while ensuring the liquid does not run over or cover the labels of bottles and other containers.
- All staff around a sterile field should wear gowns and gloves. Those working directly on the sterile field should use sterile masks.

Evaluate Infection Control Precautions Implemented by Staff Members

Nurses directly and indirectly watch out for themselves and other staff members to ensure they adhere to the right infection control and prevention measures. They can offer immediate education to staff who have not properly learned the various infection prevention procedures and can be involved in planning, designing, and evaluating the results of more organized educational activities for staff members.

Evaluate Whether Aseptic Techniques Are Performed Correctly

Aseptic techniques should be carried out in accordance with generally accepted procedures. Nurses should evaluate and monitor the process to ascertain staff members' competency and that they have correctly adhered to the procedures.

Use of Restraints/Safety Devices

Restraints and other safety devices may be required in situations where mobility can increase the risk of falls or where there is a risk of suicide or self-harm.

Assess the Appropriateness of the Type of Restraint/Safety Device Used

There are different kinds of restraints that can be used depending on the situation. The restraints include the following:

- Belts, jackets, and other devices that will prevent limb movement.
- Patient restraints that will restrict movement.
- Temporary seclusion in a room with the intent to protect the patient or others. This ensures that the patient's basic needs are met.
- Medications that may reduce agitation or aggressive behavior for a specified period under medical guidance.

Follow Requirements When Using Restraints

Ethical considerations and individual restraint requirements must be kept in mind. Heavy restraints should only be used as a last resort when other control measures are ineffective. Restraints should not be used as punishment, and restraining measures should not cause further harm to the patient.

Nurses should be trained on how to use restraints appropriately.

Patient rights and ethics must also be considered when using restraints. National and state laws on the use of restraints must be followed, and the concerns of family members of patients who are being restrained must also be acknowledged.

Patients who are under restraints must be provided with special care, as they may need assistance with activities such as moving their bowels, eating, and maintaining hygiene. Restrained patients should not remain in the same position for long to prevent cramps and bed sores. Patients who can speak and are conscious of their environment should be allowed to communicate their inconveniences so they can be properly cared for.

Lastly, all restraining procedures should be properly documented.

Monitor/Evaluate Client Responses to Restraints/Safety Devices

Patients who are under restraints should be closely monitored to prevent further harm. A restraint should be removed immediately if it poses a threat to the patient. Nurses should look out for signs, such as difficulty breathing, pallor, blue skin, and choking when restraints are used. Nurses should also periodically check for optimal blood flow and watch out for numbness, peeling, and bruises at points where restraints are attached.

Restraints should be removed as soon as it is deemed safe, considering both the patient's condition and the potential risk to themselves and others.

Chapter 2: Health Promotion and Maintenance

The Aging Process

Aging comes with challenges, and people respond to these challenges differently. It is, therefore, necessary for a nurse to identify and assess the responses of individuals to these changes and challenges as they occur.

For some toddlers, the changes associated with weaning might produce a defiant reaction. Others might have difficulties adapting to toilet training or the arrival of a younger sibling. School-aged children might have challenges adapting to school routines, and older kids might react to puberty differently.

For young adults, there are usually significant changes associated with higher responsibilities like marriage, pregnancy, and childbirth. Some adults might adopt positive coping mechanisms to cherish the journey and experience. In contrast, others might adopt maladaptive coping mechanisms that result in total disgust for their body changes and accompanying responsibilities.

Older adults must adapt to changes in their bodies as they get slower and become unable to perform all the activities they once used to. This stage can also be filled with the possibility of regrets over decisions that should or should not have been made. There is a feeling of loneliness and isolation at this stage.

Irrespective of the stage of life that clients are in, a trained nurse must assess clients' reactions to these changes quickly.

The nurse should note patients who adapt well and those with maladaptive reactions.

Providing Care and Education for Newborns, Infants, and Toddlers from Birth through 2 Years of Age

Neonates

The World Health Organization (WHO) defines neonates as newborns up to 28 days of age. Children have the highest chances of developing complications at this stage, which can result in death. Hence, the nurse must be vigilant for signs of ill health in neonates.

Since neonates cannot speak or complain, the observation skills of the nurse must be top-notch. At birth, the first assessment is the APGAR score. This is a quick way to evaluate the status of a child at birth. APGAR stands for Appearance, Pulse, Grimace, Activity, and Respiration.

- *Appearance*: The nurse should examine if the neonate is pink all around, has a pink body with bluish extremities, or is bluish all around.
- *Pulse*: The pulse should be checked to see if it is absent, less than 100 beats per minute, or greater than 100 beats per minute.
- *Grimace*: A neonate should be assessed for the presence and strength of their grimace in response to stimulation.
- *Activity*: The neonate may either be inactive with weak flexion of the arms and legs or actively crying and moving body parts.
- *Respiration*: Respiration is evaluated as either absent, slow, irregular, or good, with vigorous crying.

Each parameter in the APGAR score is assessed as 0, 1, or 2. The total is added up to 10. If a child scores 0 to 3, then the child is in severe distress and needs urgent intensive care and resuscitation. Neonates who are scored 4 to 6 are moderately distressed and require immediate attention. Neonates who are scored 7 and above are generally in good condition.

Gestational age is another parameter that is used to assess a neonate. To measure the gestational age, the New Ballard Scale is used. This scale is based on both physical maturity and the maturity of the neuromuscular system. It is graded from -1 to 5 and measures the following parameters:

- Posture, square window, which refers to the wrist's movement (varies from greater than 90 degrees to 0 degrees).
- Arm recoil (ranges from 180 degrees to less than 90 degrees).
- Scarf sign (neonate crossing arms over chest).
- Heel-to-ear movement.

The average neonate measures 18-22 inches with a head circumference of 12.5-14.5 inches and weighs 5 lbs 8 oz to 8 lbs 13 oz.

- *Vital signs*: Respiratory rate 30 to 60 breaths per minute.
- *Pulse*: 100 to 140 bpm.
- *Blood pressure*: 60/40 to 80/50 mmHg.
- *Temperature*: 97.7 to 98.9 degrees Fahrenheit.

Abdomen: Full, round, moves with respiration, bowel sounds present within a few hours of birth, umbilical site clean and free of discharge or discoloration.

Head: Head circumference within normal range, eyes bilaterally equal in size and shape. Observe eye movements. Ears should be placed at normal levels bilaterally. Low-set ears and abnormal eye and nose position can suggest Down syndrome.

The mouth should have a closed oral palate, with pi oral mucosa and bilaterally symmetrical lip and tongue movements. Observe for excessive salivation, which might indicate a tracheoesophageal fistula.

Neonate skin should be pink without sustained blueness, jaundice, or cyanosis. Lanugo hair, vernix caseosa, and telangiectatic nevi might also be present.

Fontanels should be soft and flat, with no depression or bulge. Bulging could indicate raised intracranial pressure, while depression may suggest reduced pressure due to dehydration. Molding might be present if the delivery was vaginal.

Excretory and urogenital systems: Meconium should be passed within a day of birth. Male testes should descend into the scrotum, and the presence of the prepuce covers the glans and rugae in the scrotum. Some females may have swelling in the labia and blood from the vagina.

Infants

Infants are greater than 28 days and up to one year of age. At this age, infants are in Erikson's first stage of development, the trust versus mistrust stage. At this stage, infants expect everything they need in terms of food, love, care, warmth, and security to be provided by their caregivers. If these needs are unmet, the child can develop a feeling of mistrust and that adults are not dependable.

This stage also coincides with Piaget's first phase of cognitive development in children, known as the sensorimotor stage. Children learn about their surroundings through sensory and motor activities at this stage.

What to Expect

- Suckle reflex.
- Grasping reflex.
- Moving eyes and ability to focus on objects for limited periods.
- Cooing and babbling.
- Responding to sudden movement or loud noises and some selected words.
- Doubled birth weight by six months.
- Teeth begin to develop.
- Increase in length (1 inch per month until one year).
- Increase in head circumference.
- Ability to transfer objects hand to hand (usually at about nine months).
- The child forms bonds with parents and caregivers.
- Separation anxiety sets in at this stage.
- Feeding every two hours with formula or breast milk (the WHO recommends exclusive breastfeeding for babies in the first six months of life).

Toddler (1–3 Years of Age)

Some call this developmental stage the "terrible twos" because children begin to explore and exhibit defiant behavior and tantrums.

Children at this age are now at Erikson's second stage of development, which is known as autonomy versus shame and doubt. At this stage, children are focused on the development of self-control. They often desire to expand their capabilities either independently or with assistance. At this stage, they do things impulsively, act out of curiosity, and become very energetic.

They might not like the rules set in place, as they want to do things on their own terms. This may lead to frustration, tantrums, and inappropriate behavior.

At this stage, they should learn and master potty training.

Parents and caregivers are expected to provide opportunities for the toddler to make independent decisions, no matter how small. This might be anything from selecting snacks to eat to what clothes to wear.

Providing Care and Education for Preschool, School-Age, and Adolescents from 3 through 17 Years of Age

Preschoolers (3–5 Years of Age)

This stage coincides with Erikson's third stage of psychosocial development. It is called the initiative versus guilt stage. Here, the child begins to dominate and control the world around them.

The initiative phase of this stage allows for exploration and experimentation through play. Children begin to explore the power of imagination and the freedom to create.

Failure to complete a task or overcome an obstacle can lead to a feeling of shame and guilt in children at this stage. It is a "good" versus "bad" situation for children. They are "good" if they excel in tasks and "bad" if they do not.

At this stage, children refine their motor skills. This is the stage at which disabilities affecting development are more pronounced. They usually experience an annual weight gain of four to seven pounds and an annual growth of two to three inches.

What to Expect

- Able to stand on one foot for longer than 10 seconds.
- Able to hop around.
- Draw a person with features.
- Follow simple directions.
- Decrease in separation anxiety.
- Able to express feelings and desires verbally.
- Dress and undress on their own.
- Need reassurance and encouragement always to try again if they fail at any tasks.
- Failure should not be why they do not attempt new tasks or experiences.

- Children at this stage should be allowed to take the initiative in play or explore their surroundings if it does not endanger them or others.

The School-Aged Child (6–12 Years of Age)

At this stage, the child is now at what Erikson termed the industry versus inferiority stage. Here, the child begins to learn about accomplishments and abilities. At this stage, the child begins to associate success with competence and a feeling of superiority, while failure is met with feelings of inferiority. If children are always encouraged and praised at this stage, they will develop a corresponding sense of competence and belief in themselves.

Piaget's cognitive development theory places children at this age in the concrete operational stage. They can solve problems by considering several angles, outcomes, and perspectives. They can also solve problems that have to do with conservation. Conservation is the understanding that certain properties of objects remain the same even when their outward appearance changes. Solving conservation-related problems helps with mathematical problems and word problems, which are key skills required of this age group.

What to Expect

- Challenge authority figures around them.
- Follow complicated commands.
- Perform actions that require combining several motions.
- Retain information.
- Prefer same-gender friends and peers.
- Emulate their parents of the same sex.
- Recall names, addresses, ages, best food, and personal details.
- Menarche might develop, as well as other secondary sexual characteristics.

Adolescents

The WHO defines this age group as 10 to 19 years old.

Erikson defines it as the identity versus role confusion stage. Here, teenagers develop a sense of identity. This sense of identity goes a long way in determining the type of people they will be. If this identity is well determined, the individual will usually be stable. If the teenager cannot do so, they might become confused and develop a weak sense of identity and self.

Piaget describes this as the formal operational stage, where there is much abstract thinking. Teenagers can think about abstract concepts easily, even those that are not rational or realistic. They can also apply reasoning skills to solve problems more coordinated and systematically.

At this stage, they share typical vital signs with adults. There is an increased need for calories due to the growth spurt in this stage. Completion of sexual maturity occurs in this stage.

What to Expect

- Attraction toward the opposite sex.
- Self-conscious.
- Seek peer group acceptance.

Providing Care and Education for Adults from 18 through 64 Years of Age

Young Adults

According to Erikson, young adults between 19 and 35 are at the intimacy versus isolation stage. Here, they begin to form closer, stronger relationships with other people.

What to Expect

- Seek purpose in life.
- Healthy coping mechanisms develop to deal with work demands, relationships, and other commitments.
- Preventive steps are taken to reduce the occurrence of chronic conditions as they age.

Middle Age

Middle age typically begins around the age of 40 and lasts until the age of 65. Muscular strength begins to decline. There is a reduction in sexual drive, and menopause and erectile dysfunction may occur.

Individuals in this stage are at what Erikson termed the generativity versus stagnation stage. Adults at this stage are concerned with a need to produce structures, people, and things that will outlive them. They are also concerned about their impact on the world and seek to improve the lives of others.

What to Expect

- Worries range from the care of children to the care of aging parents.
- Diagnoses of chronic health conditions.
- Concerned with legacies that outlive them.

Providing Care and Education for Adults Ages 65 Years and Over

This is the final stage of psychosocial development seen in the elderly. It is called the integrity versus despair stage. People at this point usually look retrospectively at the influence of their choices earlier in life. They either regret the consequences of their decisions, which causes despair, or find happiness in the meaning and purpose of their lives.

What to Expect:

- Gradual decline in physical function and musculature.
- Sensorineural changes: Decreased ability to see, hear, smell, and touch, slower reaction times, and night blindness.
- Cardiovascular: Reduced cardiac output, stroke volume, reduced venous return.
- Musculoskeletal: Decrease in muscle mass, muscle tone and strength, degenerating joints, bones, and reductions in intervertebral disc spaces.
- Renal: Reduction of kidney size, decreased creatinine clearance, and decreased glomerular function.

- Hepatic changes result in reduced hepatic blood flow and metabolism that causes reduced hepatic clearance and a subsequent increase in the concentrations of medications in the body.
- Skin: Wrinkling, increased skin fragility, graying of hair, dry skin, reduced turgor and elasticity, thicker nails.
- Respiratory: Reduced lung expansion, increased risk of respiratory infections.
- Fluid and electrolyte changes.
- Reminiscing over accomplishments or regrets in life.
- Increase in the occurrence of sickness and death.
- Retirement.
- Need to change the environment to adapt to needs.
- Require more assistance in performing daily activities.

Great care should be taken when medication is prescribed for older adults. This age group has a significant impairment in drug distribution, absorption, and clearance. The nurse must be conscious of this when attending to older individuals.

Pre-/Intra-/Postpartum and Newborn Care

Assess the Client's Psychosocial Response to Pregnancy

The pregnancy period places emotional demands on both parents and relatives. There are varying psychological reactions when a pregnancy is announced, whether expected or not.

Some concerns around pregnancy can include fear of body changes, financial burdens, anxiety, delivery concerns, and the safety of the fetus.

Some people have strong family support that helps them through pregnancy, while others do not.

Assess the Client for Symptoms of Postpartum Complications

After childbirth, there is a risk of postpartum complications, especially hemorrhage, if delivery is via SVD. Postpartum hemorrhage can be prevented by active management of the third stage of labor. Administer 10 IU of oxytocin immediately after delivery to contract the uterus and ensure that the entire placenta is delivered through controlled cord traction and uterine massage.

The nurse checks for malfunctions in reproductive organs, records and reports any abnormal changes, and provides nursing interventions as fast as possible. Examination of vital signs, weight, amount of blood loss, intake and output, and mental state is also important.

Assessment for the risk of vaginal, uterine, or cervical infections after childbirth is done by looking out for symptoms of fever, itching, swelling, redness, and other presenting signs.

Calculate the Expected Delivery Date

A pregnant mother is expected to know the date to anticipate when she will have her baby. This is relayed during prenatal clinics, and the nursing officer can educate mothers on estimating dates between 36 and 40 weeks of pregnancy.

For example, a pregnant woman can run ultrasound scans to determine EDDs but can also manually calculate dates using the last menstrual cycle date preceding the pregnancy.

Check Fetal Heart Rate During Routine Prenatal Exams

At the clinic, nursing officers usually educate pregnant mothers on the importance of prenatal care. This includes listening to the fetal heart rate, which can be assessed using a Doppler device or an ultrasound.

The nurse can check for signs of distress in pregnancy resulting from an increased fetal heart rate of up to 200 BPM, often associated with uterine conditions or maternal health issues such as hypertension, infections, sepsis, certain lifestyles, and medication.

Assist the Client with Learning and Perform Newborn Care

The nurse is responsible for educating new mothers on how to care for their newborns. This includes caring for a newborn through breastfeeding, bathing, umbilical cord care, diapering, and cleaning the baby's feeding items if they are not breastfed.

Also, the nurse teaches mothers how to monitor the growth and development of their children according to the developmental milestones chart.

Provide Prenatal Care and Education

Prenatal care involves health education and assessing mothers' pregnancy risks or unhealthy behaviors, such as smoking, alcohol, and stress.

Pregnant women are counseled during prenatal clinics about the importance of practicing health-compliant behaviors, especially the impact on the unborn baby's cognitive and mental state.

Diagnostic tests, blood tests to check for infections (HIV, Hepatitis B), blood sugar levels, rhesus factors, vital signs monitoring, and weight assessments are all done in prenatal care to prevent or reduce the risk of adverse events during labor.

During prenatal care and education, a mother will also be taught about nutritional needs, such as meals or supplements essential for the baby, regular clinic visits, childbirth methods, and how to deal with multiple gestation.

Provide Care and Education to a Prepartum Client or a Client in Labor

In the four stages of labor, the client is expected to be aware of presenting symptoms. The nurse is also expected to be ready for complications that can arise at any of these stages. This is highlighted to the pregnant mother with coping techniques to adopt for the safe delivery of the baby.

Nursing interventions are key at this point. The nurse provides emergency care and seeks the safety of the client. Patient hygiene, fetal heartbeat, and dilation are all checked during labor. Several delivery methods are presented to the client as appropriate. These include vaginal delivery, cesarean section, forceps delivery, and water birth.

The consequences or complications of the chosen method should also be communicated to the client, especially when there is a breech position, preeclampsia symptoms, tachycardia, or other cardiac abnormalities. The relatives are educated on the client's need for care and support.

Provide Postpartum Care and Education

Before discharge, postpartum care is given to the mother, which will enable her to handle her health and that of the newborn. The nurse is responsible for examining the client and providing adequate information about hygiene, childcare, feeding, and complications such as hemorrhage and sepsis.

Education on the care of the reproductive organs, use of analgesics, mother and child attachment, laboratory scans, and family planning methods are given to women who opt for vaginal delivery.

The client is informed on how to reach out to healthcare practitioners for further review, especially when symptoms of postpartum psychosis are suspected.

Provide Discharge Instructions (Postpartum and Newborn Care)

Before a newborn is discharged, the mother is given instructions to handle emergencies and look for noticeable changes in the baby's skin color and overall health.

Education is provided on bathing, keeping the baby warm, hygiene, and breastfeeding.

In the case of a young woman who has just had a baby and is expected to meet the demands of a paid job after a few weeks, the nurse can advise against possible stress.

Evaluate the Client's Ability to Care for the Newborn

The nurse assesses the client's ability to independently care for the newborn by observing the client perform all necessary procedures.

Observation sessions can be conducted, or role-play trials can be used to see that the client understands the necessities of newborn care, such as cleaning the umbilical cord, medication administration, circumcision, breastfeeding, bottle feeding, putting the baby to sleep, comfortable carrying, and perineal care.

Health Screening

Health screening is an essential part of health promotion and maintenance.

Apply Knowledge of Pathophysiology to Health Screening

To effectively perform health screening, nurses must be able to apply knowledge of the disease process or progression. They must be able to identify the signs and symptoms of disease progression to detect or diagnose a condition as fast as possible. They can refer clients for further investigations when an express diagnosis is impossible.

Examples of routine screening examinations that should be performed in different populations include:

- *Blood sugar*: Blood sugar can be checked while fasting (known as fasting blood sugar) and not fasting (known as random blood sugar). A fasting patient should not have a blood sugar that exceeds 100 mg/dL, but some researchers allow a reading up to 125 mg/dl. A patient's random blood sugar should not exceed 200 mg/dl. If any of these values are out of range, it indicates a need for further testing. Understanding the pathophysiology of diabetes mellitus, which could cause a rise in blood sugar, informs this screening. If the condition is diagnosed in a younger individual, it is often Type I. If the condition is diagnosed in an older individual, it is often Type II. Further tests are required to confirm the diagnosis, such as HBA1C or FLP.

- *Blood pressure*: A routine screening checks the systolic and diastolic blood pressure. The expected normal blood pressure is 120/80 mmHg. Understanding hypertension's pathophysiology, which raises blood pressure, informs this screening. Hypertension is defined as blood pressure greater than 140/90 mmHg. However, pre-hypertension stages occur before crossing 140/90 mmHg, followed by stages I and II.

Diagnosis is made after at least two readings taken at separate times are persistently above the normal values.

- *Fasting lipid profile*: A test used to diagnose high cholesterol levels. Adults should do this test at least once every five years. It detects the levels of total cholesterol.

- *Colorectal screening*: For adults over 50, colorectal screening should be done regularly. Screening for colorectal cancer in this age group is informed by understanding its pathophysiology, as it is the most prevalent among them. The screening might include colonoscopy, sigmoidoscopy, digital rectal examination, fecal occult, and blood testing.

- *Breast cancer screening*: This is very important in all women of 40 years and above. A mammogram should be done earlier for women with a family or personal history of breast cancer or a breast pathology such as a mass or lump. Several health awareness campaigns advocate for breast self-examination among women.

Perform Health History/Health and Risk Assessments

A health history is one of the most significant ways of obtaining health information from clients.

A nurse must be aware of the two classifications of data:

- *Primary and secondary data*: Primary data refers to data collected directly from the client or patient. Here, you receive the information directly. Primary data also includes data that a nurse obtains from observation or examination of the client. Secondary data is obtained from other sources, such as relatives, medical records, and other healthcare personnel.

- *Objective and subjective data*: Objective data refers to data that can be measured and observed objectively. It can be seen, felt, or touched. The inferences made from it are largely unquestionable. Subjective data cannot be objectively measured. It is based on the client's personal experiences and feelings and can be influenced by individual perceptions. A good example is pain measurement, in which a patient might describe a grade of 8/10. Another patient with more resilience and a higher pain threshold could describe the same pain as a 5/10.

Taking a detailed health history is done in an interview style. This interview can be carried out with both open and closed-ended questions. Open-ended questions allow clients to express themselves and talk freely about their complaints. For instance, "What brings you to the emergency department today?" or "What were you doing when you started feeling the headache?"

Close-ended questions are suitable for "Yes" or "No" questions. Such as, "Do you have children?" or "Are you married?"

A health history should include the complete biodata, the presenting complaints, the history of presenting complaints, and past medical and surgical history. This includes previous admissions and diagnoses, psychological, family, and social history.

Perform Targeted Screening Assessments

Routine screening is done to detect conditions that are very general to a specific group of people or the general population. However, target screening can be done when some people show strong tendencies, signs, or symptoms of a particular condition or disease. This target screening is also done when a client is at risk of a certain ailment or needs to rule out a possible condition.

For instance, a child not gaining the expected weight and not feeding well might need a nutritional assessment. A child having difficulty reading from far distances might need a visual acuity test performed. A student who begins to act withdrawn, with a loss of interest in enjoyed activities, might need an evaluation of mental status. This is not routinely done, but a targeted screening assessment can be done based on the observed symptoms.

Utilize the Appropriate Interviewing Techniques when Taking the Client's History

When interviewing clients, more than knowing how and when to use open and closed-ended questions is required. Nurses should also be aware of other essential elements that contribute to a successful interview, making obtaining information from the client easier.

- *Be open, trusting, and nonjudgmental*: No matter the condition, be open to understanding clients' perspectives, even if what they say is not correct from a professional stance. By actively listening to clients, you can identify the areas where they require more assistance.
- *Ensure confidentiality at all times*: Every patient has a right to privacy, and this includes asking questions and discussing issues that are private to them. Create an environment free of distractions so the patient feels safe and comfortable to speak. You may need to ask relatives to wait or step aside from the patient when you require information.
- *Eliminate communication barriers*: Language, for instance, might be a barrier and require an interpreter's presence.
- *Use excellent communication techniques*: Apply all the knowledge of communication that you have gathered over time. Utilize open and close-ended sentences and active listening.
- *Speak to relatives when needed*: Do not hesitate to speak to relatives when they need to be consulted over an issue. Also, when patients cannot answer questions about their health and/or they did not leave an advance directive, the relative should make that call.
- *Cross-check all data with the client to avoid errors*: Patients should always say their names in full. All data should be clearly and professionally documented.

All these techniques are essential and determine how successful the nurse is in getting the required information from the patient.

Assess Client Lifestyle Risks that Impact Health

High-risk behaviors are actions that significantly increase the likelihood of client harm, disease, or death. Most of these are modifiable behaviors that are based on choice. They can include diet choices, a sedentary lifestyle, violence, and drug abuse.

Biologically, some risks are evident based on race, age, and gender and cannot be modified. For instance, the female gender has a higher chance of breast cancer than the male gender. In the same vein, prostate cancer is seen in males. Depression is diagnosed more frequently in females, but suicide rates are higher in males. Some races have a higher propensity to certain ailments than others.

However, high-risk behaviors can be modified, either by stopping the activities altogether or replacing them. Nurses must be able to recognize behaviors that significantly impact the lives of their clients. Examples include:

- Excessive exposure to the sun.
- Sedentary lifestyle.
- Unbalanced diet.
- Cigarettes or other tobacco products.
- Alcoholism.
- Drug abuse.
- Unprotected sexual intercourse.
- Lack of sleep.

Nurses must be able to assess clients and their lifestyles to recognize high-risk behaviors that can influence their health in the short and long term.

High-Risk Behaviors

Assist Clients in Identifying Behaviors and Risks that Impact Health

Nurses must identify high-risk behaviors and guide clients to understand the harm such behaviors can cause to their health. This is mostly done through client education, where nurses must help clients recognize the unsafe practices they engage in. For instance, a man who is admitted for a case of hypertension and still engages in excessive drinking and smoking should be made to see the effects of his lifestyle choices.

Clients should be counseled appropriately about the effects of their lifestyle choices and how to change them.

Educate Clients About the Prevention and Treatment of High-Risk Health Behaviors

After pointing out the high-risk behaviors, it is the responsibility of the nurse to share practical steps that can be taken to eliminate them.

A patient having regular unprotected sex can be counseled on abstinence or condoms to reduce the risk of contracting STIs. Nurses can also counsel patients on contraception to prevent unwanted or unplanned pregnancies.

For instance, a patient struggling with smoking habits can be referred to a psychologist or therapist for help.

Some age groups have higher risks of death from automobile accidents. Nurses can advise on preventative measures such as wearing seatbelts, checking vehicle conditions before driving, and abstaining from driving under the influence.

The most important aspect is that the steps are easy to understand and implement.

Health Promotion and Disease Prevention

Health promotion is one of the core components of nursing care.

Assess and Educate Clients About Health Risks Based on Family, Population, and Community

There are several health risks that individuals are exposed to daily. These risks are based on the patients' age, socioeconomic status, hobbies, lifestyle choices, location, and population.

Individuals, families, groups, and communities are all levels of clients that can be assessed for specific needs and health risks. For instance, an individual might have an increased risk of reinfection from an unhealed wound following surgery. A family might have children at risk of malnutrition if the mother is not well informed about the benefits of a balanced diet and eating right. Populations might be at risk of a pandemic if vaccinations and immunizations are not taken seriously.

Assess the Client's Readiness to Learn, Learning Preferences, and Barriers to Learning

As important as assessing the client is, it can be tough to obtain cooperation if a nurse does not know the client's preferences and barriers.

Therefore, significant measures must be taken to understand clients. This includes how ready they are to learn, the best method for them, and possible barriers to their learning.

Readiness to learn is divided into four types:

A. *Physical readiness*: This involves the measures of ability, the complexity of the task, the effect of the environment, the health status of the individual, and gender. The measures of physical ability determine whether a patient is ready to learn. A patient with a motor impairment might find it challenging to perform fine movements and might not be ready to learn things, such as cleaning a surgical wound appropriately. The complexity of the task must be proportional to the level of individual ability. The environment and health status can also affect an individual's physical ability to learn. A patient who is still drowsy and semi-conscious will not be ready to learn anything. A patient in unfavorable conditions might not be readily receptive to lessons on maintaining a clean environment. Some studies suggest that females may display more readiness to learn certain health-related topics due to traditional caregiving roles. However, a readiness to learn is influenced by various factors and cannot be generalized based solely on gender.

B. *Mental readiness*: This deals more with the cognitive and psychological aspects of readiness. For example, a client who has just been diagnosed with a terminal condition might not be in a state of readiness to learn about it. The client might still be in shock or denial, and learning at this stage would be abortive. An anxious patient might also not be ready to learn because they cannot concentrate.

C. *Experiential readiness*: This deals with the levels of aspiration, coping mechanisms used in the past, the locus of control orientation, and self-efficacy. Locus of control refers to where an individual's control or power over the future lies. In some people, the locus of control is internal. In others, it is external. When it is internal, individuals believe they have control over their future and any trouble they might encounter. When it is external, individuals believe that the future and whatever problems they might encounter are beyond their ability and lie in an external factor, like people. The internal locus makes people more ready to learn. Self-efficacy is an individual's belief that they can achieve a task or goal. It can either motivate or inhibit learning.

D. *Knowledge readiness*: Refers to the current level of knowledge of the learner, the level of capacity to learn, and the preferred style of learning of the individual.

The style of learning varies from individual to individual. Some styles include visual learning, verbal learning, tactile (touch) learning, active learning, reflective learning, and sequential learning.

Nurses should always combine multiple learning methods when educating several people at once. However, when educating individual clients, they can utilize a person's most preferred learning method.

Barriers to Learning

The barriers to learning are many, and they depend on individuals, environments, and teachers.

- Language barriers: Individuals who cannot communicate in the primary language of the care provider or educational content may need an interpreter or translator.

- Literacy level: When the literacy level of a client is low, the client might have difficulty reading and writing as well as understanding some technical words.
- Inadequate health information can also limit learning.
- Stress or pain can also be a barrier to learning, as the client might not be open physically or mentally to learning.
- Cultural and spiritual beliefs can hinder learning, as they can make the individual close-minded to health facts.
- Physical and functional limitations such as disabilities or amputations can limit learning that requires physical movement.
- Financial limitations can also hinder learning. A client might need help to pay for a procedure, training, class, or required materials.

Plan or Participate in Community Health Education

Community health education refers to organized efforts to promote, maintain, and improve health among target populations. It involves improving the personal, community, and organizational health in society.

Nurses must provide education to achieve these objectives of developing health characteristics. This involves assessing the particular health needs of a community. When these needs are identified, the nurse can devise an intervention plan. It might involve educating community members via presentations, counseling, and guidance for individuals or even multidisciplinary cooperation. Regardless of the method, the nurse must be prepared at all times.

Evaluate Clients' Understanding of Health Promotion Behaviors/Activities and Educate Them on Actions

Health-promoting behaviors are actions that help increase individuals' health and well-being. Examples are exercise, a balanced diet, abstinence from smoking, abstinence from unprotected sex, avoiding drug abuse and illicit drugs, and receiving regular check-ups.

Assessing a client's knowledge of health-promoting behaviors can be done by asking questions. These questions can be informal but provide an understanding of the client's level of knowledge.

Assessments can be structured and formal questions. They can also be made by observing the behavior of the patient. Patients not caring about hygiene or washing their hands before eating might need to be made aware of the health implications.

Similarly, a client who does not bother about weight and continues to eat all types of junk food might either be ignorant or prefer to ignore the consequences of their actions.

Other assessment methods include focus groups, self-administered questionnaires, tests, and documentation. Once the assessment has been done, educating the patient becomes straightforward.

Weight Management

Patients can work with a fitness coach, physical trainer, and nutritionist to lose weight gradually over time. Clients can be educated about the complications of obesity and how it contributes to poor prognosis in many health conditions.

Smoking Cessation

Patients often continue to smoke even though they know the harmful effects of their actions. This can be due to addictions, depression, and maladaptive coping mechanisms. Smoking cessation will require multidisciplinary cooperation with therapists, psychologists, and physicians.

Balanced Diet

A balanced diet helps to boost the body's immunity and ensure proper growth and development. When people do not eat well, their immunity breaks down. As a result, productivity, growth, and moods are affected. Nurses might need to collaborate with nutritionists to counsel clients on eating right. Patients with diabetes also benefit from this.

Exercise

Exercise is a health-promoting behavior. Clients should be counseled against a sedentary lifestyle. The WHO recommends at least 150 minutes of moderate-intensity exercise or at least 75 minutes of vigorous-intensity exercise weekly.

After educating the patient, follow-up is necessary to ensure that the therapies and education are productive. A follow-up helps identify patients needing more help to achieve their goals.

Apart from pharmacological and clinical interventions, some forms of treatment can effectively promote health. They include alternative and complementary therapies, such as meditation, prayers, chiropractic services, music, acupuncture, or yoga.

Educate Clients on Preventative Care and Health Maintenance Recommendations

A nurse also educates clients about routine recommendations to preserve health and prevent diseases. These include screening tests and routine examinations such as:

- Diabetes screening.
- Cervical cancer screening in women.
- Prostate cancer screening in men.
- Colorectal cancer screening.
- Hepatitis B and C screening.
- HIV testing.
- Hypertension screening.
- Glaucoma screening.
- Obesity education.
- Breast examination.
- Testicular examination.
- Good nutrition and regular exercise.
- Weight management.
- Lifestyle choices such as cessation of alcohol, smoking, and substance abuse.

Provide Resources to Minimize Communication Barriers

Communication is the exchange of information between at least two people. It involves the sending and receiving of information.

A barrier to communication is anything that prevents communication from happening.

Communication barriers can include:

- *Language barriers*: If clients do not understand English, they may have difficulty understanding what the nurse says. An interpreter that understands the client's language may be needed, or translation devices can be used if available.
- *Physical communication barriers*: Communication over wider distances and spaces can be easily misunderstood. Speaking to a large audience might be ineffective when educating or counseling a patient.
  Solution: Nurses can engage a larger audience with general information while providing smaller breakout groups for clients to ask questions and receive emphasized information. In some cases, one-on-one counseling might be required, as some individuals might be too shy to speak about their challenges in front of others. Different mediums should be explored depending on the information that needs to be shared.
- *Physiological barriers*: These are barriers due to the abnormal function of a body part, such as a hearing or visual impairment. When this is the case, nurses should recommend a hearing aid or use sign language if the patient is completely deaf. If a person is blind, then Braille can be used in addition to speaking.
- *Psychological barriers*: Some patients might not be in a state of mind that is receptive to communication. A patient who just received a terrible diagnosis might be shocked and depressed. A parent waiting for a child in surgery might be anxious. Patients might also have mental health conditions that do not make them open to communication.
  Solution: Nurses should understand the time or place for communication. If a patient or client is not in the best frame of mind and the information is not urgent, it can be deferred until another time. If urgent, the nurse must be professional and empathetic while conveying the message. If it is a mental condition, then as treatment progresses, the client should be able to understand and receive information.

Other things to take note of in overcoming communication barriers include:

- *Active listening*: Nurses should listen to their patients carefully. People can tell if someone they are speaking to is listening or not.
- *Clarity*: Most clients need help understanding medical jargon. Therefore, nurses should always speak in terms that patients can understand.
- *Avoid information overload*: The patients should be given time to take information in. Other healthcare personnel might be seeing them and giving them information. Therefore, patience is required so that clients do not get overwhelmed.

Assist the Client in Maintaining an Optimal Level of Health

Nurses also have a role in helping patients to maintain an optimum level of health. An optimum level of health means the best possible health attainable by an individual based on their current health status.

For instance, a person with an amputated limb due to diabetes can still reach optimal health status by checking blood sugar and complying with drugs. The person can use an artificial limb and crutch. A nurse can also collaborate with other specialists, such as physiotherapists, to help the patient learn to balance with the artificial limb or crutches.

Nurses can provide counsel on foot examination and prompt reporting to the health facility in case of any wound or break in the skin of the viable limb. They can counsel on wound care at the surgery site and the flap created at the amputation site. They can also teach the client about signs of infection, such as pus, foul smell, discoloration, or persistent bleeding.

Lifestyle Choices

Assess Clients' Lifestyle Choices

Apart from the lifestyle choices discussed in previous sections, other choices greatly affect the health status of individuals. The other decisions include relocation to urban or rural areas, the decision to send children to public or private schools, and career decisions. All of these significantly affect the health status of individuals and families. For instance, for parents with remote work and flexible schedules, nurses may notice a difference in how they interact with their children compared to those who are out of the house most of the day. This difference can be observed in the relationship between the children and their parents and the amount of attention paid to their diet, growth, and academic performance.

Assess Clients' Attitudes and Perceptions of Sexuality

A nurse must be able to assess a patient's views and beliefs about sexuality. This includes sexual orientation, perception of gender, contraception, premarital sex, and sexual partners.

Nurses must remain impartial and professional when relating to patients with different sexual orientations and perceptions, irrespective of their beliefs.

Assess Clients' Needs and Desires for Contraception

Some clients might decide they do not need contraception. Nurses must be unbiased about the choices that each patient makes. They must share the benefits and disadvantages of different contraception types, including abstinence, withdrawal, calendar method, barrier method (male and female condoms, diaphragm, cervical cap), injectables, implants, intrauterine devices, female sterilization (bilateral tubal ligations), and pills.

Identify Contraindications to the Chosen Contraceptive Method

Some contraceptive methods have contraindications.

- *Transdermal patches*: History of smoking cigarettes, heart disease, deep venous thrombosis (DVT), breast cancer (or other estrogen-related cancers).
- *Diaphragm*: History of latex sensitivity.
- *Combined oral contraceptive pills (COCP)*: History of smoking cigarettes, heart disease, DVT, breast cancer (or other estrogen-related cancers).
- *Emergency contraception*: Known or suspected pregnancy.
- *Vaginal rings*: History of smoking cigarettes, heart disease, DVT, breast cancer (or other estrogen-related cancers).

Identify Expected Outcomes for Family Planning Methods

Some of the expected outcomes of using contraceptives are:

- Ability to plan pregnancy.
- Ability to prevent unwanted pregnancy.
- Ability to have a satisfying sexual life without pregnancy concerns.
- Ability to select the best methods of contraception based on needs and personal choices.

Recognize Clients Who Are Socially or Environmentally Isolated

When individuals are isolated, there are many implications for their health. It can result in depression, suicidal thoughts, low self-esteem, and feelings of rejection. A nurse must be able to identify any individual who feels socially or environmentally isolated. This can be due to age, sickness, relocation of family members, or death of a spouse.

Once the client is identified, interventions can be planned.

Educate Clients on Sexuality Issues

Clients must be educated on sexuality issues depending on their stage of life.

The primary concern for those of childbearing age is fertility and family planning. Fertility can be an issue for either the man or woman. Infertility can be due to hormonal changes, infections, sexual dysfunction, trauma, or surgery. Medical advancements and tests can help, which include in-vitro fertilization and medical and surgical interventions.

Evaluate Alternative or Homeopathic Healthcare Practices

The alternative health industry has risen in recent years, with a surge in demand for natural remedies.

Homeopathy uses a natural approach to combat sickness and disease. Although the effectiveness of some homeopathic remedies is not fully established, the FDA has regulated them. However, this does not necessarily mean that all homeopathic products are safe or effective.

Self-Care

An ultimate self-care plan covers physical, emotional, psychological, spiritual, financial, and environmental needs.

Assess the Client's Ability to Manage Care in the Home Environment and Planning Care Accordingly

Assessment is a unique function of nurses. An ultimate self-care plan covers physical, emotional, psychological, spiritual, financial, and environmental needs.

This plan includes identifying basic activities of daily living for the client to manage after discharge. Activities of daily living include personal hygiene, environmental sanitation, feeding, moving around, relationships, shopping, exercise, and identification of certain medications to be used.

Most times, patients being managed for mental disorders, certain illnesses, or disabilities are assessed for their willingness and ability to care for themselves. Nurses check for physical strength, neurological balance, eye coordination, and movement. They enforce resources or aids to advocate for wellness and swift recovery.

For instance, a middle-aged man who was involved in an accident and lost the use of both lower limbs can be taught by the nurse how to care for himself. Assessment of the client's need for a wheelchair, assistance with mobility, assistance with bowel movements, and maintaining oral health are some ways to ensure functional independence.

Similarly, caring for a client who recently underwent colostomy surgery involves proper hygiene assessment and monitoring of personal intake and output.

Consider the Client's Self-Care Needs Before Developing or Revising the Care Plan

Clients' needs are unique, and nurses must approach them as such. Then, an existing care plan can be modified based on need, or a new plan can be established.

For example, managing bowel movements differs from personal hygiene self-care reviews.

Chapter 3: Psychosocial Integrity

Psychosocial integrity refers to equilibrium in the psychological and social areas of life. A nurse must be aware of factors that affect these areas and how to intervene when necessary.

Abuse or Neglect

Assess Clients for Abuse or Neglect and Report, Intervene, and Escalate

Abuse refers to any action that intentionally causes harm to another person. There are several types of abuse:

- **Physical abuse:** This is the most recognized and involves any action that physically harms or injures another person, such as hitting, slapping, punching, confinement, unwilling isolation, force-feeding, and unauthorized restriction of movement.
- **Sexual abuse** refers to any form of sexual contact without consent. It can include unwanted touching, rape, and forced nudity.
- **Emotional abuse** refers to causing emotional or mental pain deliberately.
- **Neglect** refers to depriving a vulnerable adult of basic or essential care needed to help maintain physical or mental health. Neglect can be due to actions or inactions, including failure to provide food, water, shelter, medications, or access to healthcare.
- **Exploitation** refers to the illegal use of a vulnerable individual's resources for another person's profit. This can include illegally withdrawing money from a person's account, forcing a person to provide money, or stealing items from a person.

The nurse must be able to identify signs of abuse.

Signs of physical abuse include bruises, black eyes, open wounds, untreated injuries, repeated visits to the hospital with injuries and lacerations, caregivers refusing to allow visits to the vulnerable adult, and reports of physical assault.

Signs of sexual abuse include bruises around reproductive organs, unexplained vaginal bleeding, shredded, stained, or bloody undergarments, reports of sexual assault or rape, and unexplained STIs.

Signs of mental abuse include personality changes, emotional agitation, anxiety around specific persons, reports of verbal or mental mistreatment, unusual behavior, withdrawal, and nonresponsive behavior.

Signs of neglect include malnutrition and poor personal hygiene, bed sores from lying in the same position, reports of maltreatment, dirty clothing, and unsafe and unhygienic living conditions.

Once these factors are identified, the nurse must report and plan interventions as appropriate.

Identify Risk Factors in Domestic, Child, and Elder Neglect and Sexual Abuse

Some of the risk factors for abuse include:

- Older adults with cognitive impairment.
- Children with developmental problems.
- Mentally disabled people.
- Physically disabled people.
- History of mental health disorders in the abuser.
- History of substance use with the abuser.
- Poor anger management skills of the abuser.
- Crisis in the family or at work.
- Individuals with no source of income or limited education.
- Previous history of abuse.

Plan Interventions for Victims or Suspected Victims of Abuse

Planning interventions can only be done after thoroughly assessing the patient's needs. Once this assessment is done, the nurse should prioritize meeting the patient's needs.

The needs to be met depend on the presentation of the client. Patients who present with open wounds or injuries from battery should have their wounds attended to.

Malnourished people should be placed on a diet plan to supply appropriate nutrients. If a child is not feeling well, they should be nursed back to health.

Cases of abuse should be reported as the law requires.

The nurse must establish an open, trusting, and nonjudgmental relationship with the abused. Abuse victims tend to share their experiences when they feel secure and not vulnerable to exploitation.

Nurses should be able to ask questions skilfully and patiently to obtain accurate answers. It is also essential for them to be aware of the appropriate time and place for asking certain questions. For instance, a nurse may need to request the caregiver or parent of a little girl to step out of the room when asking sensitive questions.

Intervention might mean taking the child into custody. The plan might also require multidisciplinary management, such as social health services, psychologists, counselors, physicians, and nutritionists.

Counsel Victims or Suspected Victims of Abuse and Their Families on Coping Strategies

Emotional support is required for individuals going through any form of abuse, and nurses are trained to provide just that.

Because of the cycle of violence and abuse, victims might feel they need to return to the abusive relationship. They usually need reinforcement and counsel on separating from the abuser to prevent the cycle from continuing. Doing this takes time and requires much support.

The abuser should seek help, such as anger management counseling. However, the law must be involved if the abuser has committed a crime.

Abuse is a grave issue and must be treated as such. It must be handled tactfully and professionally.

Provide a Safe Environment for the Abused or Neglected Client

In the hospital, the abused should feel safe and secure. Suppose the nurse observes anxiety in the patient when someone visits. In that case, closer attention should be paid, and the visitor should not be allowed to see the victim without supervision (or possibly at all).

Abused children and neglected elderly are relocated to safe facilities determined by authorities after discharge.

Evaluate Clients' Responses to Interventions

After interventions are carried out, they should be evaluated. Was the wound well treated? Has the malnourished or dehydrated elderly patient begun to feed well? What is the client's current health status? Is the person adapting well to the new home they have been moved to? How well is the child coping with the situation?

Behavioral Interventions

Behavioral interventions aim to modify the behavior of individuals. Nurses must identify patients who require them.

Assess Clients' Appearance, Mood, and Psychomotor Behavior and Respond to Inappropriate or Abnormal Behavior

Nurses can gauge a patient's psychological status by using appearance, mood, and psychomotor behavior. These provide good insight into the mental health status of the individual.

A nurse should observe the patient's appearance to identify any signs that are indicative of possible conditions. A patient who dresses inappropriately for the weather, such as wearing thin clothing during the winter, might be struggling with a psychological or physiological issue. The patient's gait, movement, and grooming should also be observed.

Mood can be assessed by observing both verbal and nonverbal communication. Is the mood appropriate for the occasion? A patient who begins to laugh after receiving the news of the death of a loved one needs attention.

Depression can present with low mood and loss of interest in previously enjoyed activities. This depressed mood can be reflected in the movement of the individual, which might be slow, with slumped shoulders and certain behaviors like avoiding eye contact.

Inappropriate behavior can be subtle, pronounced, or harmful to others. It is, therefore, the duty of a nurse to assess a patient properly and take proactive steps.

A patient who comes in drunk and staggering might be dangerous to themselves and others. A patient's angry outburst can upset other clients and health personnel.

A nurse should quickly inform security whenever she feels that the safety of any patient or personnel on the ward is at risk.

Assist Clients in Developing Strategies to Decrease Anxiety

Anxiety is the root of various inappropriate behaviors. Training clients to handle anxiety can be a very effective way to eliminate those inappropriate behaviors.

Coping strategies include cognitive reframing, deep breaths, progressive relaxation, prayer, meditation, music therapy, and medication.

Incorporate Behavioral Management Techniques When Caring for a Client

There are several techniques that nurses can use to help patients gain self-control over their behavior.

Preventive measures include relaxation techniques, trigger and stressor avoidance, consistent routines, exercise, alternative medicine, therapy, and socializing.

If a patient exhibits challenging behavior, the nurse may need to use de-escalation techniques. These techniques may include calmly asking the patient to stop the behavior, setting clear boundaries, or using physical restraints as a last resort to protect the patient or others from harm. Maintaining appropriate eye contact during the process can help establish a connection with the patient, but it's essential to gauge each patient's comfort level as sustained eye contact may not be comforting for everyone.

Other techniques that can be used include role modeling, in which nurses demonstrate appropriate and acceptable behavior around patients and staff members, and positive reinforcement, which involves acknowledgment and praise. Nurses should serve as accountability partners and provide support throughout the treatment.

Patient orientation is a program that helps to increase patients' sensory awareness and perceptions of reality.

Group therapy involves therapy with other people who have similar challenges. It can be grouped by age and sex.

Evaluate Clients' Responses to the Treatment Plan

The effectiveness of any plan depends on how well the patient has adhered to the structures and set goals.

These goals are the foundation for the treatment plan assessment. Common goals include demonstrating appropriate behaviors, avoiding triggers, maintaining boundaries, and participating in required therapy sessions.

Assess Clients' Reactions to the Diagnosis and Treatment of a Substance-Related Disorder

Substance abuse is the excessive use of substances, whether they are legal, illegal, prescribed, or not prescribed.

Substance abuse can lead to physical dependence, which happens when a person begins to experience adverse physical reactions upon drug withdrawal. These adverse physical effects are usually more apparent when the drug withdrawal is abrupt. However, it is important to note that addiction can occur without physical dependence.

Addiction is the constant need to take a particular substance despite physical, mental, social, or economic harm.

Psychological dependence happens when a person continues using substances to prevent unpleasant feelings.

Assess Clients for Substance Abuse/Toxicities and Intervene as Appropriate

The nurse needs to observe clients and their reactions when they are diagnosed. Some clients might be defensive, while others might feel ashamed.

Some clients might immediately admit their problem and then seek a way out. Others might blame others and rationalize their behavior. Some might present with low self-esteem masked with a buoyant personality or aggression.

Clients might have a low pain threshold, a high tendency to take risks or self-medicate, suicidal ideations, and concurrent mental disorders.

Physically, hyperactivity or sluggish movements, tremors, poor hygiene, needle marks on the upper and lower extremities, and poor health may occur.

Clients might exhibit drug-seeking behavior, such as claiming their medications have been exhausted, falsifying prescriptions, and always having an ailment that requires medication.

They might also have problems in other areas of life, such as relationships and academics.

Examples of standard tests for assessing such clients include:

- Drug abuse screening test.
- Addiction severity index.
- The CAGE-AID test.
- Michigan alcohol screening test.

Plan and Provide Care to Clients Experiencing Substance-Related Withdrawal or Toxicity

Substance-related toxicity occurs when a substance is taken in amounts that are harmful to the patient, regardless of whether it has a therapeutic dosage. Substance-related withdrawal symptoms occur when an individual cannot access a substance they have been abusing.

Some common signs of withdrawal and toxicity include irritability, restlessness, agitation, poor concentration, hallucinations, and visual disturbances.

Patient care goals for substance-related withdrawal or toxicity include:

- Safety and protection from self-harm and harming others.
- Prevention of falls.
- Relapse prevention.
- Management of physical symptoms.
- Medication should be strictly taken as prescribed.
- The family and friends of the patient are educated.
- Self-help groups that can provide support during treatment.

Educate Clients on Substance Use Diagnosis and Treatment Plan

Once a plan is designed, the nurse is responsible for explaining and educating the client on the diagnosis, treatment, and plans. The patient should be educated about viewing substance abuse as an illness, not a defect. They should also be taught how to deal with the stigma associated with substance abuse and recognize the risk factors involved.

Provide Care and Support for Clients with Non-Substance-Related Dependencies

Addictions are not limited to substances. There are non-substance-related addictions, such as sexual addiction, pornography addiction, and kleptomania.

Impulse control counseling and therapy could be helpful for clients in this category. Cognitive-behavioral therapy and drug therapy can also be beneficial in addressing these disorders.

Evaluate Clients' Responses to a Treatment Plan and Revise It as Needed

Evaluating a client's response helps determine if the client is progressing or suffering a relapse.

Some things to be considered include:

- Achieving sobriety.
- Participating in therapy.
- Responding to medication.
- Attending support groups.
- Understanding relapse and prevention mechanisms.

Coping Mechanisms

Coping mechanisms refer to patterns of behavior, thoughts, and feelings that an individual uses to maintain a stable psychosocial status whenever there is stress or a disturbance. Stress can be due to many events, such as birth, death of a loved one, jobs, or parenting.

Assess Clients' Support Systems and Available Resources

Different clients react to stress in different ways. A nurse must understand this while assessing them.

How people cope with stress is also affected by their environment and the people they surround themselves with. There are two standard assessment tools for this:

1. Interval Follow-Up Evaluation.
2. Range of Impaired Functioning Tool.

Assess Clients' Ability to Adapt to Temporary and Permanent Role Changes

Some life events have temporary effects, while others bring permanent changes.

Temporary changes can include an injury or fracture that takes weeks or months to heal. They can also include the loss of a job, with the chance of obtaining another one later.

However, permanent changes can include losing a loved one or a permanent lack of ability to perform at work.

Assessment is based on how people perceive their current status and their strategies to maintain their psychosocial homeostasis during the stressful period.

Assess Clients' Reactions to a Diagnosis of Acute or Chronic Mental Illness

Individuals react differently under stress. When the stress comes from acute or chronic illness, whether personal or that of a loved one, it can be very strenuous.

Some common psychological changes associated with acute or chronic illness include distress, anger, denial, guilt, grief, rationalization, or depression.

Assess Clients' Ability to Cope with Life Changes and Providing Support

To better understand clients' perspectives and the factors affecting their reactions, two models can be used:

- *Social and cognitive models* emphasize that clients should remain as independent as possible and be allowed to gain mastery over the situation rather than being pitied or looked down upon.
- *Nagi's model* emphasizes that disability is a function of the social environment's expectations and the client's inability to meet them.

Support could include the encouragement and teaching of the following:

- Positive self-talk.
- Reinforcement of social support systems.
- Relaxation techniques.
- Stress management skills.
- Realign and readjust goals as necessary.

Identify Situations That May Necessitate Role Changes for a Client

Some roles in life come with profound changes that need some level of adaptation. Examples are young adults with newly established family units, new parents, middle-aged adults, and those experiencing health decline. Older adults may experience limitations in capacity and chronic illnesses.

Provide Support to Clients with Unexpectedly Altered Body Images

When clients experience amputations or burns, their body image can alter, which affects their perception. When this image is impaired, it can cause them to avoid or hide the affected body part, have negative feelings and remarks about the body, or make frequent referrals to their past body image.

Nurses can:

- Allow clients to express their feelings about the alteration freely.
- Facilitate the development of a more realistic body image.
- Focus on strengths and abilities rather than weaknesses.

Evaluate Clients' Constructive Use of Defense Mechanisms

Defense mechanisms are behaviors that people employ to avoid stress.

Some of these include:

- *Displacement* occurs when a client transfers anger, aggression, or feelings of frustration at one person to another person or object.
- *Regression* occurs when a client is under extreme stress and begins to display behaviors that do not fit the person's current stage of development.
- *Compensation* occurs when a person succeeds exceptionally well in one activity or field to compensate for another area of failure.
- *Intellectualization* occurs when a person seeks to rationalize a stressful event in a way that makes it less painful or traumatic.
- *Sublimation* occurs when a client transforms unacceptable urges and feelings into socially acceptable activities or behaviors.

Other defense mechanisms include dissociation, rationalization, undoing, identification, or minimization.

Evaluate Whether Clients Have Successfully Adapted to Situational Role Changes

If a client is adapting well and receiving treatment, there are some parameters to be checked:

- Copes with situational role change.
- Realistic and achievable expectations.
- Dependence on others.
- Participation of family and friends in support and care.
- Objective or subjective signs and symptoms.

Crisis Intervention

A crisis is a time-limited event when an individual is pushed beyond their coping mechanism's limit.

There are different types of crises:

- *Developmental/maturational crises*: Predicted occurrences that happen in life. They occur due to growth (a new job or promotion), marriage, childbirth, or retirement.
- *Situational crises*: Events that are unexpected and unpredictable. Examples are severe illnesses, job loss, or the death of a loved one.
- *Adventitious crises*: Events due to a significant social disturbance, such as natural disasters, war, or terrorism.

Assess the Potential for Violence and Use Safety Precautions

There are four primary levels of a crisis that a nurse must assess for:

1. *Level 1*: Patients become anxious about life events and resort to coping mechanisms.

2. *Level 2*: Patients begin to show signs of impairment or loss of function. To cope, clients begin to use different coping mechanisms from what they were using before.
3. *Level 3*: Patients begin showing signs and symptoms of typical general adaptation syndrome.
4. *Level 4*: Patients begin to feel isolated, detached, and overwhelmed. Patients might begin to entertain thoughts of violence toward themselves and others.

The risk factors for self-harm and suicide include a history of depression, a history of self-harm, past suicide attempts, and feelings of hopelessness.

Identify Clients in Crisis

Some things to look out for include saying goodbyes, oral or written suicidal statements, a loss of interest in activities once found pleasurable, changes in personality or appearance, changes in sleep patterns, and self-harm.

Nurses should be trained on strategies to prevent violence and suicide.

Use Crisis Intervention Techniques to Assist Clients in Coping

Any threats of suicide or violence should not be handled lightly. Patients can be constantly observed, and restraints can be used if necessary. However, the first step is to establish trust with clients so that they can freely speak and express their feelings.

Then, therapy can begin, and treatment will involve strong social support in the form of family and friends, who will provide positive reinforcement.

Clients should also be taught to develop coping mechanisms and engage in individual and group therapy. Nurses should educate them about their conditions, identify signs of relapse, and effectively reach out for help when needed.

Guide the Clients to Resources for Recovery from the Crisis

Clients should be provided with resources about their condition and how they can be helped. Observe for certain outcomes such as reduced anxiety levels, the adoption of effective coping mechanisms, and an increased willingness to seek help.

Cultural Awareness and Cultural Influences on Health

Culture is the way of life of a group of people. It refers to a set of established beliefs and ideologies that a group holds and has been passed down from one generation to the next. A nurse must understand the patient's culture and its impact on how they receive care.

Assess the Importance of Clients' Self-Reported Culture/Ethnicity When Planning and Providing Care

Culture affects the way clients receive care. It affects how they perceive nurses and healthcare workers. A nurse must know how to relate to clients without offending their cultural beliefs.

Leininger's transcultural nursing theory proposes a model for both universal and specific nursing care. It proposes three nursing models that nurses must understand in order to provide care for people of different cultures:

- Cultural preservation and maintenance.
- Cultural care negotiation and accommodation.
- Cultural care repatterning and restructuring.

These models provide a balanced approach to assessing culture and how it affects the delivery of care.

Incorporate Client Cultural Practices and Beliefs When Planning and Providing Care

Nurses must always allow for their clients' cultural practices and beliefs when they provide care. Many times, this determines if the care will be received or rejected.

Some areas in which people hold different beliefs include:

1. *Perceptions about health and sickness*: Some cultures believe that ill health is a stigma, so they distance themselves from it. Some promote health-seeking behavior. Others do not believe in medical care or believe in rituals and alternative medical practices.

2. *Attitudes towards healthcare professionals*: A client might not readily receive intervention from a nurse. A nurse must patiently and tactfully introduce the concept of care. Such clients must not be rushed.
3. *Family dynamics*: The structures of families differ from culture to culture. Some cultures allow only males to make decisions about the family, including health matters. Others allow equal sharing of such responsibilities. Some cultures require the oldest member of the extended family to make decisions on behalf of other family members. A nurse must know who to approach when decisions are to be made.
4. *Self-efficacy*: Some cultures believe people can change their destinies or fate. Hence, they are willing to take steps to protect their health. Individuals with other cultural beliefs may not be motivated to take steps because they believe the outcome depends on fate.
5. *Space and proximity*: Some individuals are used to living in small towns with few people and might have difficulty adjusting to a busy hospital setting.
6. *Communication*: Cultures heavily influence communication patterns, which affects both verbal and nonverbal communication. A nurse might need an interpreter or translation device. A nurse must also be conscious of gestures, eye contact, and signs that might be offensive to a patient.

Understanding these areas will help the nurse relate better with clients of different cultures.

Respect Clients' Self-Reported Cultural Background and Practices

No matter how different a culture might seem, a nurse must respect all cultures as long as the particular beliefs do not harm clients.

Evaluate and Document How Client Language Needs Were Met

Documentation is part of the process of evaluation and growth. A nurse should document how client needs were met despite cultural differences and the techniques that worked. This not only helps the client to receive better care but also helps other nursing staff members to provide care in a way that the person understands.

Particular attention should be paid to the client's level of comprehension, compliance, and adherence to care and treatments. Documentation of client accommodations, including instructional materials, interpreters, and translation devices, is important.

End-of-Life Care

End-of-life care can be challenging for everyone involved because of the physical, mental, and emotional strain. However, nurses must remain calm because the clients need them to be at their best during such periods.

Assess Clients' Ability to Cope with End-of-Life Interventions

A nurse must be able to assess the ability of a patient to cope with end-of-life interventions. A patient at this point has needs that are different from routine patients. They need physical, psychological, spiritual, and social care.

Physical needs include adequate nutrition and fluids due to anorexia and dehydration. There might also be a need for pain medication.

Patients might have psychological needs. They might battle with confusion, sleep disturbances, fear, and depression. These fears might result from different things, such as what will become of the family after they are gone or fear of the unknown. The nurse can correct some of these issues, while others might have to be managed with the help of psychologists and family members.

Assist Clients in the Resolution of End-of-Life Issues

End-of-life care should be adequately provided for clients that need it. In addition to what was mentioned earlier, this care might include proper hygiene, ensuring the patient is comfortable, and providing privacy. It also includes proper turning and positioning of the patient at regular intervals, massage, and therapy.

Provide End-of-Life Care and Education to Clients

Nurses should educate clients about what to expect at this stage. The families and support system of the client should also be educated about the signs and symptoms to expect toward the end of life. Legal documents and advance directives must be sorted out so that there are clear instructions on what to do and what not to do after death.

Family Dynamics

Different patterns influence the outlook of life of family members, including their perspective on healthcare. The patterns determine how authority flows in the family, who makes the decisions, who is the leader, and who is responsible for the care in the family.

Assess Barriers and Stressors That Impact Family

Several barriers can impact the function of the family unit, including:

- *Physical*: Food, housing, or transportation.
- *Biological*: Ill health, disability, or death.
- *Socioeconomic*: Unemployment, underemployment, or financial losses. Behavioral factors: Lifestyle choices like drinking, smoking, or substance abuse.
- *Societal factors*: War or civil unrest.
- *Cultural and spiritual factors*: Acceptance or rejection of a specific culture by children. They may make different lifestyle choices than what is expected.

All these factors affect the function of the family in one way or another. Barriers such as lack of funds, lack of needed transportation, and lack of cohesion in the family can all affect healthcare.

Assess Parental Techniques Related to Discipline

Some parents are liberal, and others are strict. Some go as far as abuse, and nurses must be sensitive to know when a child is being abused. When violence is involved, nurses must report it to the appropriate authorities.

A nurse must observe all family members, especially the dependents, for signs of depression, withdrawal, or isolation, as these can all point to abusive behavior from the parent or caregiver.

Encourage Clients to Participate in Group or Family Therapy

Many families might not be open to family therapy. Nurses must be able to educate the family members on the need for group therapy and its benefits.

Assist Clients in Integrating New Members into the Family Structure

A new member of a family can be a stressor. This can be a problem in some families, especially if dysfunctions exist. A nurse can provide education on what to expect from a new family member. In the case of a new infant, the parents and siblings should be prepared on what to expect and how to care for their newest family member.

Evaluate Resources Available to Assist Family Functioning

After assessing the family's state, the nurse can provide resources to aid the family. This can be anything from educational materials to resources in the community and referrals to qualified personnel who can provide therapy for the family.

Grief and Loss

Grief is a normal response to loss, which can cause emotional, physical, social, and intellectual reactions. Individuals eventually learn to accommodate or live with the loss.

Every loss will impact clients directly or indirectly, and the extent of grief that they exhibit will vary from person to person.

There are several types of grief, including:

- Dysfunctional grief.
- Anticipatory grief.
- Cumulative grief.
- Collective grief.

Provide Care for Clients Experiencing Grief or Loss

To properly provide care for a grieving patient, the nurse must understand the stages of grief. There are several theories with different stages.

The most popular theory is the *Kübler-Ross model*, which describes grief in five stages:

I. *Denial* is when the person refuses to accept the loss that has occurred.
II. *Anger* can be directed at oneself, the family, friends, or the world.
III. *Bargaining* involves wishing things could return to what they were before the loss. It might also involve bargaining with a higher power if the event can be avoided.
IV. *Depression* is when the person begins to feel a profound sense of grief. It is an essential stage in healing.
V. *Acceptance* involves living with the new reality that the person is gone.

Other models include *Sander's Phases of Bereavement*, which include shock, awareness of loss, conservation, withdrawal, turning point, and renewal.

Worden's Four Tasks of Mourning include accepting the loss, working through the pain of grief, adjusting to a world without the deceased, and finding a way to remember the deceased while moving on with life.

Engel's Stages of Grieving involve shock and disbelief, developing awareness, restitution, resolution of the loss, idealization, and outcome.

A nurse must understand what stage clients are in and help them accordingly. The first step is to establish trust so the client is open to receiving help.

The nurse should also educate clients about coping strategies. There might be a need for referrals to social or religious groups. The services of psychologists might also be needed.

Standardized tools such as the *Hogan Grief Reaction Checklist* and the *Texas Inventory of Grief* can be used to assess clients for complicated grieving.

Support Clients in Anticipatory Grieving

Anticipatory grief begins before the event happens. It is usually seen in terminal illnesses or amputation of a body part.

The nurse can provide education on what to expect while being as gentle and empathetic as possible. However, the facts should not be withheld or watered down, as this can negatively affect the client's expectations.

Inform Clients of Expected Reactions to Grief and Loss

Nurses should inform clients of what to expect while grieving. It might not be the happiest news to hear, but it helps to know that at least the nurse understands them.

Evaluate Clients' Coping Mechanisms and Fears Related to Grief and Loss

Clients must be evaluated to see how well they have coped with grief and loss. They should be expressive about their feelings and not withdrawn or isolated. They should seek help and have effective coping mechanisms to resume their everyday lives in one year or less.

If a client does not focus on anything but the loss and cannot move beyond it, the patient might be experiencing complicated grief and require further help.

Mental Health Concepts

Mental health is pivotal in treatment and care. Nurses must know about mental health disorders, how to assess them, and what interventions are required.

Recognize Signs and Symptoms of Acute and Chronic Mental Illness

A nurse must recognize the signs and symptoms of a mental illness, whether acute or chronic.

Some mental illnesses include:

1. **Depressive Mental Health Disorders**: These include major depressive disorder, dysthymia, and postpartum depression. Tools for assessing this group of disorders include the *Beck Depression Inventory*, the *Geriatric Depression Scale*, and the *Hamilton Depression Scale*.

Signs and symptoms include low energy, depressed mood, sleep loss, poor judgment, weight loss, anorexia, libido loss, personality changes, low self-esteem, hallucinations, delusions, suicidal ideation, and suicide.

2. **Anxiety Disorders**: These include generalized anxiety disorder, various phobias, panic disorder, acute stress disorder, PTSD, and obsessive-compulsive disorder. Tools for assessment include the *Yale-Brown Obsessive-Compulsive Scale*, the *Modified Spielberger State Anxiety Scale*, and the *Hamilton Rating Scale for Anxiety*.

Signs and symptoms vary with specific disorders. Phobias present with anxiety or stress due to a particular object, event, location, or situation. Panic disorders present with chest pain, severe anxiety, difficulty breathing, and palpitations. Generalized anxiety disorder presents with persistent and prolonged worry over various situations. OCD presents with such things as pathological hoarding.

3. **Bipolar Disorder**: This presents with intermittent episodes of mania, hypomania, and depression. Signs and symptoms include elevated mood, irritability, depressed mood, restlessness, loss of inhibition, increased sexual drive, loss of sleep, and grandiose delusions.

4. **Cognitive Mental Disorders**: This includes dementia and delirium. Signs and symptoms include difficulty reading, poor writing and speech, inability to recognize people or places, and poor short-term memory. Behavioral changes and impaired processes might also be present.

5. **Personality Mental Disorders**: These can be grouped into different clusters. Cluster A includes schizoid, paranoid, and schizotypal mental disorders. Cluster B includes narcissistic, antisocial, histrionic, and borderline disorders. Cluster C includes dependent and avoidant personality types. Signs and symptoms are dependent on the type of personality disorder. Cluster A personality disorders generally display odd or eccentric behavior. Cluster B personality disorders generally display dramatic or erratic behavior. Cluster C personality disorders are typified by anxious or inhibited behavior.

6. **Eating Disorders**: These include anorexia nervosa, bulimia nervosa, and binge-eating disorders.

Anorexia nervosa: It is characterized by the excessive limitation of food intake, extreme fear of weight gain, irritability, amenorrhea, and low body weight. Some individuals with anorexia may engage in binge-eating and purging behaviors, but these are not defining characteristics for all cases.

Bulimia nervosa: Binge eating rapidly, followed by purging.

Binge eating: Repeatedly consuming large amounts of food at once.

7. **Psychotic Disorders**: These include schizophrenia, schizotypal personality disorder, and schizoaffective disorder. Signs and symptoms include:

Cognitive symptoms include poor attention and concentration, poor judgment, and impaired decision-making. Affective symptoms include depressed mood, feelings of dejection, suicidal thoughts, hallucinations, delusions, and lack of energy and motivation.

8. **Substance Abuse and Addictive Disorders**: These include alcoholism, sexual addiction, and pornography addiction.

Provide Care and Education for Acute and Chronic Psychosocial Health Issues

Nurses are responsible for providing care for people with different behavioral health issues. Some of these issues might be acute, while others might be chronic.

The basis of providing care is the establishment of trust. Clients must be able to express themselves to the nurse freely. With this, a nurse can begin to provide the necessary care.

The care here would involve maintaining a safe, therapeutic environment for the client, administering prescribed medication, counseling, continuously observing the patient's mental status by assessing behavior, and educating the client and family members.

A nurse should educate the client and family members about the cause of the disorder and its triggers and flashpoints. A nurse should also discuss relieving factors, such as individual therapy, group therapy, drugs, and follow-up care.

Evaluate Clients' Ability to Adhere to the Treatment Plan

Some clients might adhere to the treatment plan provided by the healthcare team, while others may not. A nurse must evaluate the client's adherence to the plan.

Some of the parameters to look out for include the willingness and participation of the client in the plan, previous experiences where a similar treatment plan did not work, lack of insight of the client, the judgment of the client, denial, self-efficacy, internal locus of control, and side effects of the plan.

Religious and Spiritual Influences on Health

The influence of religion on a person can be powerful. Hence, a nurse must understand how religion and spiritual beliefs affect health.

Assess Psychosocial Factors Influencing Care and Plan Interventions

Several psychosocial factors influence the planning and delivery of care.

Occupational factors can include the nature of the job and the work hours. Some occupations may only allow patients the time to visit the clinic on weekends. Thus, a nurse must create a flexible schedule for patients with such time constraints.

Other factors may pertain to remote workers who sit for long hours in front of a laptop. They must be educated on the need for antiglare glasses and regular breaks. They must also be counseled on needing a comfortable chair and working environment to prevent back pain or complications in the future.

Spiritual or religious factors play key roles in the planning and delivery of care.

There are many branches of Christianity, including Catholicism and Protestantism. Some Christians have beliefs about fasting, communion, and newborn baptism.

Judaism also has different sects, some of which believe in circumcision, a kosher diet, and death rituals.

Hinduism has philosophies and practices such as yoga, a strictly vegetarian diet, and death rituals.

Islam forbids pork and alcohol. Some Muslim women choose to wear veils that may cover part of their faces, but this is not a universal practice. Islamic funeral practices often involve wrapping the body in a plain white shroud.

Jehovah's Witnesses do not believe in blood transfusions, eating foods containing blood, abortion, or suicide.

A nurse must attend to patients with a consciousness of their spiritual leanings and provide appropriate, respectful care.

Sensory and Perceptual Alterations

Sensory and perceptual alterations usually occur at specific times, places, and when the client is exposed to certain stimuli. Identifying where patients are most vulnerable to these alterations can help prevent or reduce them.

A nurse should help the client develop coping mechanisms for these alterations or disturbances.

Provide Appropriate Care for Clients Experiencing Visual, Auditory, or Cognitive Alterations

Patients experiencing visual, auditory, and cognitive impairments are at risk of inflicting harm on themselves and others. They can display aggressive or violent behaviors. Hence, appropriate care must be provided for them.

For patients experiencing auditory hallucinations, medication is usually the mainstay of treatment. Medication can also be combined with psychotherapy, education on coping mechanisms, and cognitive-behavioral therapy.

Patients experiencing visual hallucinations usually have an underlying disorder such as schizophrenia. The underlying disorder should be treated, and medication can also be used. Cognitive-behavioral therapy and psychotherapy can also be helpful for patients with this condition.

Provide Care in a Nonthreatening and Nonjudgmental Manner

Nursing care for patients with alterations or perception loss must be provided nonjudgmentally, no matter their behaviors.

Provide Reality-Based Diversions

Clients not oriented in time, place, or person can be helped by creating reality-based diversions and activities. Activities include discussions and taking a walk.

Stress Management

Homeostasis refers to a steady state of the body and its processes. It is a state of equilibrium and is what each system of the body strives to attain.

Stressors are factors that disrupt the equilibrium of the body. They can come in different forms, such as physiological, psychological, physical, emotional, or spiritual.

Hans Selye proposed the general adaptation syndrome, which divides the body's response to stress into three stages:

- Alarm.
- Resistance.
- Exhaustion.

Recognize Nonverbal Cues to Physical or Psychological Stressors

For nurses to effectively manage stress, they must be able to recognize nonverbal cues and respond appropriately. To do this effectively, nurses should understand the three stages of Selye's theory.

Alarm is the stage where specific physiological responses occur due to a perceived threat. Here, the patient might experience an increased heart and respiratory rate, along with higher levels of adrenaline and cortisol. These responses are the body's way of preparing for a 'fight or flight' reaction.

The *resistance* stage is marked by increased cardiac output, a maintained respiratory rate, and increased blood pressure. Here, the body is trying to deal with the effects of stress. If it succeeds, the body will return to its normal resting mode. If not, it continues in this resistance stage for a while before moving to the third stage.

The third stage is *exhaustion*. At this point, the body has used all its resources to deal with the stress. If this stage is not reversed, morbidity and mortality may result.

A nurse must learn how to look out for the mentioned signs. Other signs to watch include loss of consciousness, hyperglycemia, and hypoglycemia.

Provide Information to Clients on Stress Management Techniques

A nurse should educate clients on stress management techniques, which include daily exercise, massage therapy, meditation, and music therapy.

Therapeutic Communication

Therapeutic communication refers to exchanging information between patients and healthcare givers using verbal and nonverbal cues that prioritize clients' emotional and psychological well-being.

Use Therapeutic Communication Techniques

A nurse must be able to use different means of therapeutic communication to reassure and counsel patients. Some of these techniques include:

Active Listening involves listening carefully to the patient, processing the information, and observing the client's nonverbal communication.

Silence is a powerful tool of communication that, when properly utilized, can allow some time to process and deliberate before giving a response. However, this silence must not be prolonged so the client does not feel the nurse is not interested.

Open-ended questions aid in gathering comprehensive client information and facilitating conversation.

Paraphrasing is a good way for nurses to show they are following a conversation. It helps to clarify things. For instance, "Do you mean that the pain you felt yesterday is not as severe as what you feel today?"

A nurse must be able to focus the discussion on the important issues at hand while still acknowledging the client's feelings or concerns. A client, for instance, might begin to discuss how he misses his pet. A nurse can respond, "It sounds like you really miss your pet. Let's also discuss your hypertension and how we can address it."

Clarification can be done by restating, paraphrasing, and reflecting on the client's words.

Nontherapeutic communication techniques to avoid include:

- *Challenging*: This means forcing clients to defend their choices and opinions.
- *Probing*: This is an invasive way of gathering information and is uncomfortable for clients.
- *Changing the subject*: This can be perceived as rude or uninterested in what clients say.
- *Defensiveness*: This involves a nurse defending her own beliefs or opinions.
- *Disagreeing*: A nurse should try to educate clients therapeutically and not argumentally.
- *Judgments*: A nurse must be nonjudgmental at all times.
- *Stereotyping*: This should always be avoided.

Encourage Clients to Verbalize Feelings

Once trust is established between a nurse and a client, it becomes easy for clients to express how they feel verbally.

Therapeutic Environment

Creating a therapeutic environment that facilitates and promotes the recovery of patients is essential to nursing care.

Evaluate Clients' Use of Stress Management Techniques

A nurse must evaluate how much progress is being made by clients in terms of stress management.

Identify External Factors That May Interfere with Client Recovery

Factors that can interfere with client recovery include family stressors, weak support systems, inaccessibility to quality healthcare, and social stigma. Internal factors such as comorbidities and patient cooperation can also influence recovery.

Make Client Room Assignments That Support the Therapeutic Milieu

Assigning rooms to clients should be done to support creating and promoting a therapeutic milieu. A client who has suicidal tendencies, for instance, should be kept where nurses can observe the patient.

Promote a Therapeutic Environment

The goal of every nurse must be to establish and promote a therapeutically conducive environment for all patients. This type of environment is referred to as the therapeutic milieu.

This environment includes rules, boundaries, appropriate behavior, consistency, and client expectations.

Chapter 4: Physiological Integrity

Physiological integrity is divided into four components:

a. Basic care and comfort
b. Pharmacological and parenteral therapies
c. Reduction of risk potential
d. Physiological adaptation

Basic Care and Comfort

Basic care and comfort includes assistive devices, mobility/immobility, nonpharmacological comfort measures, nutrition, oral hydration, and postmortem care.

Use of Assistive Devices

Assistive devices are pieces of equipment used to improve, augment, and maintain an individual's performance and overall well-being. Assistive devices related to mobility and walking include walking canes, walkers, crutches, wheelchairs, and prosthetic limbs. Other devices such as alerting devices, sound amplifiers, electronic amplifiers, and hearing aids are designed to aid hearing loss. Patients with visual disabilities of any form may use corrective glasses (concave and convex) and magnifying glasses.

Assess clients for actual or potential difficulty with communication and speech, vision, and/or hearing problems.

Basic care and comfort of patients begins with an assessment of communication, speech, and visual acuity difficulty. Patients may have actual or potential speech, hearing, and vision difficulties. Patients may be referred to an ophthalmologist and audiologist for further diagnosis.

Cerebrovascular accidents such as a stroke can affect areas of the brain that deal with speech (speaking and understanding). These patients need a great deal of attention in addition to their use of assistive devices. People who are on medication such as certain antibiotics that are ototoxic may eventually need assistive devices.

These drugs damage the ear and may cause initial symptoms of tinnitus and vertigo (ringing in the ear).

Elderly patients are also predisposed to macular degeneration in their eyes, which may result in total or partial blindness. Patients with chronic conditions such as diabetes can end up with visual complications such as blindness. Some medications including antihistamines and antipsychotics can have ocular side effects. Nurses should know these types of patients and keep an eye on them.

Assess the clients' use of assistive devices.

It is the nurses' responsibility to assess the patients' use of devices and educate them on the correct use.

Assist the clients in compensating for a physical or sensory impairment.

A patient with a traumatic accident and a movement disability may need to use a walking cane. The cane should align with the patient's height for proper movement. The cane should be adjustable to permit the patient's elbow to flex slightly. The patient holds the cane opposite to the leg that needs support. For example, if the left leg is weak, the patient will hold the cane in the right hand.

Other patients use wheelchairs. There are manual wheelchairs that need the patient to apply upper arm strength to move them or an assistant to push the chair. All of these assistive devices should be maintained and cleaned appropriately.

Patients may need special equipment to maintain their personal grooming. For example, patients may need adaptive hairbrushes, combs, and special nail clippers. Also, oversized clothes, socks, and zipper pulls may help some patients, along with certain kinds of toothpaste and toothbrushes.

Patients with assistive devices are prone to further accidents and injuries. Nurses should educate patients and their relatives on home care to prevent further complications.

Elimination

Urinary elimination is a normal physiological process. After the ultrafiltration of plasma and selective absorption and reabsorption, urine must be eliminated from the body as it contains waste products, harmful metabolites, and toxic substances.

Assess and manage clients with alterations in bowel and bladder elimination.

Urine elimination can be estimated in terms of quantity. A patient may eliminate urine above the normal reference range for a period of time. This is called polyuria. Polyuria can be caused by renal diseases, diuretic medication, and diabetes mellitus. Other symptoms that can result from urine elimination quantity are reductions in urine output below the standard reference range for some time, oliguria, dysuria, urinary incontinence, urgency, and urinary frequency. These symptoms hint at the pathology in the body and the urinary system.

Fecal elimination is also a normal physiological process. Fecal elimination follows the normal absorption of food and the digestion of food and nutrients. Pathologies that can affect fecal elimination include fecal impaction, which is the collection of hardened stool in the rectum. Constipation and some medications can also cause fecal impaction. Flatulence is the expulsion of malodorous gastrointestinal gas. Flatulence can be caused by foods or medication.

The knowledge of urinary and fecal elimination and their pathologies will help a nurse assess and manage patients with such illnesses. Some patients are highly predisposed to having urinary and fecal elimination problems. For instance, a patient on diuretics for heart failure or edema may have polyuria and an excess quantity of eliminated urine. Other patients who eat foods with high salt or sodium content may actually have more excretion of urine due to the body's attempt to eliminate excess sodium. Elderly male patients may have difficulty with urine elimination because of an enlarged prostate. For other patients, a structural defect or anomaly may be responsible for problems with urine and fecal elimination. It is also important to note that urine and fecal elimination are multifactorial, as they can be structural, functional, and even psychological.

Management of patients with urine and fecal elimination may require intervention by a nurse. Interventions such as proper positioning during micturition and defecation are simple. Exercise to promote bowel movement is a simple intervention. Some patients only need privacy and comfort to empty their bowels and bladder. Food and diet also help improve bowel movement and fecal elimination. Foods such as boiled lentils, black beans, and split peas contain high fiber and help promote bowel function.

Medical management of elimination problems includes the use of pharmacological agents to relieve elimination problems. It is usually attempted before surgical interventions. Medication can improve urine elimination. Such medications include oxybutynin and darifenacin. Medical management of constipation includes enemas. Enemas are fluids that are introduced into the rectum to stimulate the emptying of the bowels. Although they can be used for constipation, they are not used as treatments for fecal incontinence or flatulence.

Urinary catheterization is a minor surgical procedure to relieve urinary retention and empty the bladder. Nurses should be careful with this procedure as it can introduce microbes directly into the genital tract if it is not aseptic. Once the catheter is placed in situ, ensure that the urine bag is emptied as necessary.

Another form of surgical management is colostomy. A colostomy is a surgical procedure that creates an opening (stoma) from the colon to the surface of the abdomen to divert fecal content. There are different types of colostomies, all with a similar goal of allowing proper elimination.

The overall aim of these interventions, whether therapeutic, medical, or surgical, is to restore and improve the elimination capacity of the urinary and rectal tracts.

Evaluate whether the clients' ability to eliminate is restored or maintained.

Restoration of elimination function and capacity is accompanied by the ability to perceive voiding clues. Also, the patient will be free of symptoms such as urinary urgency, frequency, and pain. The absence of diarrhea and constipation is a sign of restored eliminating function. Patients who show positive signs that normal urinary or bowel functions are restored may be evaluated and possibly discharged.

Mobility/Immobility

Nurses should understand why and how immobility can occur in patients.

Assess clients for mobility, gait, strength, and motor skills.

Mobility is the ability to move freely and with purpose. The first skill a nurse should have in managing patients with potential immobility is assessing gait and movement. Just like most disease conditions, risk factors predispose people to stiffness. These factors can be genetic or acquired. Genetic factors may contribute to conditions like spasticity, but cognitive impairment and the natural weakness of bones and muscles are not solely genetic. Some other patients acquire immobility due to medication use, overdose, malnutrition, impaired gait, and trauma.

When a nurse identifies patients with these risk factors, the next step is to assess for actual immobility. Assessment of mobility begins with observation. For instance, a patient with a weak gait could become immobile. Nurses can also assess immobility in a patient by giving simple instructions. For instance, ask the patient to move on the bed or around it. Assessment of mobility also involves the time it takes for the patient to get up from the seat. The ability to sit on a chair and to stand is also part of mobility assessment.

Mobility is multifactorial. The nerves, muscles, electrolytes, and psychology all come together to ensure proper mobility. Any of these can be affected so mobility is compromised. Muscle contraction is one of the parameters that determine proper mobility. It can be assessed and scored for each patient. A patient is scored from 0 to 5.

Identify complications of immobility.

The complications of immobility are systemic. It affects not only the muscular system but also the urinary, gastrointestinal, and respiratory systems.

Prolonged immobility can cause the pooling of respiratory secretions, which increases the risk of respiratory infections, atelectasis, and hypostatic pneumonia. The decreased movement of the chest and diaphragm, and the inability to effectively cough contribute to these complications. Shallow respiration and decreased respiratory movement are also complications of immobility.

When urinary muscles cannot expel urine, urine retention and stasis occur. Stasis and urine retention cause a patient to form renal stones and develop urinary tract infections.

The gastrointestinal system is also affected by immobility. Bowel movement is reduced. The patient may have constipation, impaction, and difficulty with evacuation.

Immobile skin can break down and lose its turgor. The skin of immobile patients is at risk of ulceration and may lose its strength.

Lastly, the musculoskeletal system suffers greatly from immobility. The muscles, bones, and joints become very weak. Immobility can increase the risk of osteoporosis. There's a higher risk of bone fractures. The joints can become stiff and very painful. This can further limit the patient's range of motion.

Evaluate the clients' intervention responses to prevent complications from immobility.

For the urinary and gastrointestinal systems, ensure adequate fluid intake. Fluid intake eases and helps bowel and bladder movement. Regular exercise can stretch weak muscles, bones, and joints. Also, engage the patient in deep breathing and coughing to clear the respiratory system of secretions.

Perform skin assessment and implement measures to maintain skin integrity.

The skin is the body's first line of defense. Thus, it must be well-assessed for color, odor, drainage or exudates, texture distribution, and margins.

The best way to maintain the integrity of the skin is to prevent a breakdown in the first place. Here are steps to take to prevent skin breakdown:

- Screen clients for possible skin breakdown on a regular basis.
- Always keep clients clean and dry to prevent the buildup of moisture.

- Give clients a balanced diet and adequate fluids to keep them well-hydrated and nourished.
- Use devices such as wedges, pressure-relieving mattresses, waterbeds, and pillows to prevent bed sores from friction and pressure.
- Regularly turn patients who cannot turn independently.
- Identify those clients at risk of pressure ulcers. This can be done using screening tools such as the Braden scale.

Apply, maintain, or remove orthopedic devices.

Orthopedic devices serve various purposes in skin and musculoskeletal care. Here are some of the most common:

- Traction uses physical force to exert pressure on a body part. Types include skin traction, skeletal traction, or manual traction.
- Splints are used in limb fractures to prevent further damage to the soft tissues.
- Braces are used to provide support to body parts.
- Casts are used to immobilize body parts when a fracture has occurred.

Implement measures to promote circulation.

Measures to promote circulation include the use of anti-embolism stockings and compression devices. They also include range-of-motion exercises, positioning and repositioning workouts, routine exercise, and mobilization. The goal of all these activities is to prevent the formation of clots, encourage smooth blood flow, and increase overall wellbeing. Some of these workouts also improve mental health and balance.

Nonpharmacological Comfort Interventions

Interventions and therapy can be medical (pharmacological) or nonpharmacological. Although it is crucial to know pharmacological therapy, foundational knowledge of nonpharmacological therapy is also essential.

Assess clients for pain and intervene when appropriate.

Before these interventions can be applied, patients must be assessed and diagnosed.

Acute pain is a classification of pain that is usually of short duration, (less than six months). It is rapid in onset, localized, and most likely severe. Chronic pain, on the other hand, persists beyond the typical healing time, which is usually longer than six months. Some types of pain are deep in the body and some are superficial.

Recognize complementary therapies and identify potential benefits and contraindications.

There are many nonpharmacological interventions that have potential benefits. Some are complementary, alternative, or integrative modalities. They include meditation, magnets, prayer, homeopathy, chiropractic services, acupressure, massage, and guided imagery.

Some indications for these services are chronic lower back pain, stress, neck pain, depression, and fibromyalgia.

Some contraindications to chiropractic services include acute fractures, severe osteoporosis, and certain types of spinal cord injuries or conditions. Clients with pacemakers, defibrillators, or insulin pumps should avoid strong magnets.

Provide nonpharmacological comfort measures.

Nonpharmacological comfort interventions begin with education about the patient's pain. Other comfort interventions include companionship, exercise, and massage. Distraction from their current medical condition can work well for children. Counseling sessions, drama, art, and music are other nonpharmacological interventions.

Nutrition and Oral Hydration

Nutrition plays a significant role in health.

Evaluate clients' nutritional status and intervene as needed.

Assessment of patients' nutrition can be done by collecting data. This data will include height, weight, body mass index (BMI), and waist circumference. Other data, which include laboratory values of essential chemicals such as hemoglobin, lipids, and proteins in the body, will reveal excess or reduced values. The nurse should also ask patients about their daily diet.

Managing patients with nutritional problems depends on the patient's condition. Patients with obesity should be put on a weight reduction regimen. This may include changes in diet habits and light exercises. Patients recovering from a physical disease may need to gain weight. Such patients can be put on supplements.

Provide client nutrition through tube feedings.

Tube feeding is also known as enteral nutrition. It involves passing tubes from the nose to the stomach or intestine. Clients who require tube feeding are typically those with gastrointestinal disorders, swallowing problems, burns, or any other condition that results in an inability to obtain adequate calories or nutrients through oral ingestion.

Tubes can be placed either noninvasively or invasively, although noninvasive tubes are preferred. Nasogastric tubes, which are a type of noninvasive tube, are more safely placed in patients who have an intact gag reflex and swallowing ability to reduce the risk of aspiration.

Clients should be seated 30 degrees upright. Tube feedings can be given on a continuous, intermittent, or bolus basis.

Tube placement can be confirmed by radiography, auscultation, or identifying the pH of aspirate. Input and output should be monitored, and a securing tape should always be used. The nurse should also watch out for signs of irritation, infection, or dislodgement.

Evaluate client intake and output and intervene as needed.

Intake refers to all the foods that are consumed by a patient, including IV fluids and tube feeds. Output refers to the elimination of food and fluids from the patient's body. Intake includes all of the foods and fluids that are consumed by a patient, while output refers to elimination such as urine, feces, and other bodily fluids. Urinary output is measured, and the consistency and volume of stools are noted.

Deficits should be corrected by increasing fluid intake either orally or intravenously. Fluid loss should be minimized where possible.

Personal Hygiene

Personal hygiene is the most basic care that individuals can give themselves.

Assess clients' performance of daily activities and assist when needed.

Personal hygiene should be done daily. The role of a nurse in ensuring personal hygiene includes education and assessing a patient's hygiene.

Personal hygiene starts with bathing to cleanse the body of dirt, sweat, and chemicals. Nurses can bathe patients who are in the hospital. The water temperature must be checked and soap must be available.

Other aspects of personal hygiene include perineal care, wherein the skin of the perineum is cleaned and washed regularly to avoid infections and odors. Shaving is also a part of personal hygiene. Oral hygiene involves brushing the teeth twice a day and rinsing the mouth. Nail and foot care is also part of personal hygiene.

Performing postmortem care

After a client's death, all medical equipment should be removed, such as any catheters or IV lines. The entire body of the deceased is washed and limbs are placed in proper alignment. Eyes and mouth are shut and the patient is wrapped in a shroud. The body should be identified before being transported to the morgue.

Rest and Sleep

Insomnia is the inability to sleep. It is multifactorial. Insomnia can be a result of medications except for sedative medications because they usually promote sleep. It can also be caused by the environment, illnesses, emotional and psychological disturbance, and lifestyle.

Assess the clients' sleep or rest patterns and intervene as needed.

Nurses can assess their patients for sleep patterns. For instance, while alcohol might initially induce sleepiness, it can later disrupt sleep and lead to a disturbed sleep pattern. It is also essential to record sleep patterns, such as how long the patient slept and the duration of sleep.

Pharmacological and Parenteral Therapies

Pharmacological therapies involve medications that can be taken through various routes (including orally). Parenteral therapies specifically refer to non-oral routes of drug administration. Nurses administer medication orally, intravenously, and/or intramuscularly. Parenteral drug administration refers to any non-oral method, but it usually involves injecting directly into the body, bypassing the skin and mucous membranes. Medication is a big part of the treatment regimen for many disease conditions. The knowledge of pharmacology, medication side effects, and allergies will be helpful for every nurse.

Identify adverse effects, contraindications, side effects, and/or interactions.

Medication administration requires the nurse to use critical-thinking abilities, professional judgment, pathophysiology, and detailed knowledge of patients and their conditions.

Before administering medications, the nurse must be thoroughly informed of the medications' contraindications and the patient's condition. Some general contraindications to medications include pregnancy, allergy to the medicine, and renal disease. These patients will need special considerations during drug administration and treatment.

Some drugs interact with other medications. Thus, nurses must be careful when administering multiple medications.

Some patients are allergic to certain medications. For example, some patients react negatively to medication containing sulfur. Some patients are also allergic to penicillin and antibiotic drugs called cephalosporins. Allergic reactions to drugs vary from moderate to severe and life-threatening. Nurses must assess patients to detect the possibility of reactions to medications. The signs and symptoms of allergic reactions can range from itching, body rash, swelling, and redness to reduced blood pressure, respiratory distress, and rapid pulsation.

Nurses who assess that a patient has had a severe side effect or adverse reaction from medication or parenteral therapy must record this information immediately. The patient should stop taking the drug until the doctor who prescribed it responds with further instructions.

Blood and Blood Products

Blood is a body fluid that contains plasma and blood cells. The blood cells include red blood cells, white blood cells, and platelets. Blood transports oxygen, nutrients, hormones, and waste products. It forms clots (to prevent blood loss), fights infections, and helps regulate body temperature.

Blood products are therapeutic substances derived from blood. The different blood products and their components are made of red blood cells, platelets, fresh frozen plasma, albumin, clotting factors, cryoprecipitate, and whole blood. Blood cells, especially red blood cells, have antigens. Type A blood has A antigens; type B has B antigens; type AB has both A and B antigens; and type O has neither A nor B antigens.

Individuals with blood types A, B, AB, and O can receive type O blood, but only individuals with type O blood can give type O blood to all other blood types. Patients with type O negative blood are universal donors, but they are not universal receivers. Each blood type also contains antibodies, sometimes known as agglutinins. B agglutinins are present in type A blood; A agglutinins are present in type B blood; no antibodies or agglutinins are present in type AB blood; and A and B agglutinins are present in type O blood.

Patients with hypovolemia brought on by bleeding, anemia, or other conditions involving a deficiency in coagulation or another blood component are advised to receive blood transfusions. However, people with certain religious beliefs will not accept blood transfusions.

Administer blood products and evaluate clients' response.

Before a blood transfusion, the nurse must crosscheck if the patient is the right patient. The nurse should insert a catheter and attach an intravenous line (either central or peripheral). When administering blood or a blood product, the nurse must closely watch the patient for signs and symptoms of a potential problem. When a reaction or complication is possible, the nurse must immediately halt the blood or blood product delivery.

Some complications associated with blood transfusion include febrile reactions, hemolysis, allergic reactions, and sepsis. The most common reaction to blood and blood product administration is a febrile reaction. Although a febrile response can occur with any blood transfusion, it is most commonly linked with packed red blood cells and is not followed by hemolysis. This transfusion reaction is characterized by fever, nausea, anxiety, chills, and warm, flushed skin.

ABO incompatibility, which results in hemolysis, is an incompatibility between the recipient's and donor's blood types. This incompatibility may result from a practitioner error while examining the blood and matching it to the patient's blood type, or a laboratory error regarding typing and crossmatching. The presence of flank discomfort, chest pain, restlessness, oliguria or anuria, respiratory distress, brown urine output, hypotension, fever, hypotension, and tachycardia are signs of this condition. Hemolysis is treated by administering normal saline once the transfusion is discontinued and changing all tubing to prevent kidney failure and circulatory collapse.

A blood transfusion may also cause a mild-to-severe allergic response. A blood plasma protein allergy often causes a mild allergic reaction, but a significant antibody-antigen interaction usually causes a severe one. Itching, pruritic erythema, swelling of the lips, tongue, or pharynx, as well as flushing of the skin, are symptoms of mild allergic reactions. Chest pain, low oxygen saturation, unconsciousness, flushing, shortness of breath, and respiratory stridor are symptoms of severe allergic reactions. Corticosteroids and antihistamine drugs are used to treat mild allergic reactions, whereas supplemental oxygen and pharmaceuticals are used to treat severe allergic reactions.

Central Venous Access Device

A central and peripheral venous access device can be used for venous access. When patients have accessible and usable veins, peripheral intravenous devices can be used for short-term intravenous therapy, which include fluids, electrolytes, medicines, and chemotherapy. Various factors should be considered when choosing a vein for a peripheral intravenous device. The distal veins on the non-dominant hand are the ideal choice, so the client can fully use the dominant hand. A mastectomy side, a paralysis side, or a dialysis access device is not used.

Locations distal to past phlebitis or infiltration sites should be avoided. Hand veins are not the first choice for venous access but can be used if more proximal veins are not accessible. The upper extremities are used whenever possible, rather than the legs, to avoid lower extremity phlebitis and embolism.

Insert a peripheral intravenous catheter by locating a suitable vein first and positioning the tourniquet three or four inches above the vein on the patient's arm. After cleaning the area with an alcohol swab, have the patient create a fist. Insert the catheter into the vein at a 15- to 30-degree angle. When blood flashes back into the catheter, advance the catheter a little more and then remove the needle, leaving the catheter in place. Secure and stabilize the catheter with care. Monitor and maintain the intravenous line and the insertion site after the catheter is implanted to ensure that it is patent and the flow rate is as specified. Examine the intravenous site for symptoms of infection and infiltration.

Access and/or maintain central venous access devices.

Central venous catheters are placed into the right atrium of the heart via the superior vena cava. They can be introduced into the superior vena cava through a peripheral vein, as with a peripherally inserted central venous catheter (PICC), or through the subclavian or jugular vein. Central venous catheters are the preferred method of gaining venous access when a patient is receiving intravenous fluids or treatments at home, when there are insufficient peripheral veins for the patient's needs, or when the patient is receiving therapy such as total parenteral nutrition, chemotherapy, blood, and medication.

Infection, pneumothorax, hemothorax, thrombosis, and emboli are some risks connected with central venous catheters.

When central venous lines are set, nurses must provide extra care for such patients. Central venous catheter dressings should be changed according to facility policy or at least every 7 days. Each catheter's lumen may be flushed with heparin or normal saline depending on the facility's guidelines to ensure the patency of the tubes.

Dosage Calculations

Nurses administer medications and must know how to calculate the correct dosage to avoid drug overdose.

Perform calculations needed for medication administration.

Calculation of medication dosages can be pretty technical. There are different methods for measurement and calculations. Units of measurement may differ, but a nurse should know some standard measurements. Here are a few examples:

1 teaspoon = 5 mL

1 tablespoon = 15 mL

1 cup = 16 tablespoons

1 pound = 16 ounces

1 scruple = 20 grains

1 pint = 16 ounces

1 quart = 2 pints

10 centimeters = 1 decimeter

Numbers can be written as fractions or mixed numbers. Fractions can be proper or improper. The number on top is the numerator. The number below is the denominator.

Mixed numbers are a combination of whole numbers and fractions. They should be converted to improper fractions before they can be used in calculations.

Decimals are expressed using a decimal point.

These forms of measurement are converted from one to the other. For example, when a doctor recommends a prescription in grains (gr) and you have the medication, but it is measured in terms of milligrams (mg), you will need to convert between the two measurement systems.

Calculating doses and solution rates requires nurses to use their clinical judgment and analytical skills. A nurse should be able to see an inaccurate calculation right away. Accuracy is vital in pharmacological measures because it can affect the patient's treatment. For example, medication for pediatric patients needs extra accuracy in dosage, routes, and concentration.

Expected Actions/Outcomes

Nurses anticipate outcomes from the treatment regimens of patients.

Evaluate clients' use of medication over time.

In a world where change is constant, nurses provide continuous care. The number of new medications, side effects, and outcomes is vast, which make it challenging to remember them all. As a result, nurses who administer medication must be knowledgeable about their patients' health concerns and the complexities of the medicine they use through problem-solving, clinical decision-making, and critical-thinking skills.

Some patients take pharmaceuticals for a short time for an acute sickness, whereas others are given medications for an extended amount of time for a chronic health issue. Prescription pharmaceuticals, over-the-counter medication, vitamins, supplements, and alternative medications are examples of these medications.

Evaluate client responses to medication.

Nurses caring for patients on multiple drugs for an extended period must keep track of the patients' adherence and compliance with their drug schedules. They must also assess the medication's predicted outcomes. Nurses must closely watch for adverse reactions, interactions, or undesirable effects. They must monitor patients for evidence of any accumulated effects of the drugs they've taken over time.

The term "side effects" refers to unintended consequences of a drug that are not the primary desired therapeutic impact of the medication. Some side effects can be significant. An adverse effect is a severe side effect that can sometimes be fatal, such as an allergic reaction to a medication.

Medication Administration

Medication administration is a cardinal aspect of nursing care and patient treatment.

Educate clients about medications.

Before medication administration, the patient should be informed about the medication, its expected effects, and its potential side effects. Patients, as well as significant partners, should be educated on all aspects of their drugs.

Participate in the medication reconciliation process.

The patient should know how and where the drug should be safely stored. The nurse should explain the significance of verifying the medicine's label for its name, dose, expiry date, and the method for administering it. Particular directions should be provided, such as shaking the drug, taking it with or in-between meals, or on an empty stomach.

Handle and maintain medication in a safe and controlled environment.

Some patients may need to administer medication at home. The patient should be instructed on how to self-administer drugs properly. In addition to the instructions outlined above, some patients may need to be trained on unique procedures such as using an inhaler, mixing insulin, giving oneself an intramuscular injection, or self-administering tube feedings.

Routes of drug administration include oral, sublingual, topical, transdermal, inhaled, and intravenous. The oral route of drug administration is the most common, most accessible, and most convenient for patients. The intravenous route has 100 percent bioavailability. This means that all the medication administered into the veins will enter the circulation directly.

Evaluate appropriateness and accuracy of medication orders for clients.

Nurses are responsible for reviewing every order to determine its accuracy and appropriateness relative to the patient in question.

Some of the factors to be considered include the completion of the medical order, accuracy of the order, any client allergies, the health status of the client, and significant laboratory findings.

Pharmacological Pain Management

Pain alerts the nervous system that something is amiss. It is a sensation such as a prick, tingle, sting, burn, or ache.

Administer medications for pain management.

Nurses help manage pain by administering medication to patients. The level of pain and type of pain will determine the medication dosage and the strength of the pain medication.

Analgesics are pain medications. They are broadly classified as weak, moderate, or strong. Opioids (narcotics) are used to treat moderate-to-severe pain. Non-opioids are non-narcotic analgesics that can be used as adjuvant painkillers in addition to treating mild pain. Nonsteroidal anti-inflammatory drugs (NSAIDs) are examples of non-opioid drugs.

Handle and administer controlled substances within regulatory guidelines.

It is necessary that nurses follow the required guidelines when administering controlled substances because of the prevalence of addiction and substance abuse. Here are some of these guidelines:

- Sign before receiving medication.

- Deliver the narcotics sheet to the nursing care unit along with the drugs.
- Lock drugs in secure locations.
- Count narcotics at the start and end of every shift.
- Sign upon removal of any controlled substances from the locked cabinet for administration to clients.

Total Parenteral Nutrition

Proper nutrition is associated with stronger immune systems, safer pregnancies and deliveries, a decreased risk of noncommunicable diseases (including diabetes and cardiovascular disease), and longer life spans.

Administer parenteral nutrition and evaluate client response.

Total parenteral nutrition, known as hyperalimentation, is administered through a prominent vein, such as the subclavian vein. Hyperalimentation can meet all dietary requirements, with feedings containing minerals, electrolytes, vitamins, amino acids, and trace elements that are supplied through the hyperalimentation catheter, which the physician surgically implants.

Total parenteral nutrition is used for patients who cannot or should not get their nutrition through eating. It is often used for patients who require complete bowel rest, those in a negative nitrogen balance due to conditions like severe burns, and those with serious medical illnesses such as cancer or AIDS/HIV.

Reduce the risk potential.

Reduction of risk potential is an important skill every nurse should have. It reduces the likelihood of clients developing complications or health problems related to existing conditions, treatments, or procedures.

When nurses attend to patients for a particular condition, complications may arise from disease conditions or the treatment modality. These complications are unexpected and adverse outcomes that can disrupt the patient's recovery process. They can alter the recovery process of patients and result in constant changes in the treatment regimen of patients.

Causes of complications are multifactorial. They may arise from a weak immune system or late presentation to the hospital. Complications may arise from inadequate dosing or improper monitoring of the treatment process.

Some of these factors are beyond the nurse, but nurses must make the treatment process as standardized as possible.

Notice changes or abnormalities in vital signs.

A patient's vital signs reveal much about the recovery process, status, or underlying medical conditions. A nurse should be able to assess and respond to changes in a patient's vital signs. A patient's vital signs include blood pressure, pulse rate, respiratory rate, and body temperature. These four signs signify some of the body's most basic functions. For example, a consistently high body temperature in a three-year-old child is a cause for concern.

Knowledge of the anatomy of the body and the pathophysiology of diseases is critical in noticing and responding to abnormal vital signs. For instance, knowledge of anatomy helps a nurse read the radial pulse on the lateral side of the wrist. The nurse puts the cuff around the arm to measure blood pressure. The nurse listens to the Korotkoff sounds over the brachial artery in the antecubital fossa with a stethoscope. Blood pressure readings also reveal much about what is happening to the heart. The systolic pressure indicates the force that the heart pumps blood out with and how much resistance it is overcoming.

Assessment of the respiratory rate starts by inspecting the rising and falling of the chest. An unexplained increase or decrease can be a sign of pathology in the body. For example, a decreased respiratory rate can indicate central nervous system depression. A patient who presents a reduced respiratory rate may be an opioid drug user or may have recently been overdosed with sedative drugs, which depress the central nervous system.

Conduct diagnostic tests.

Investigations are the second line of assessment in diagnosing and treating diseases. A nurse should be able to perform basic diagnostic tests. These tests reveal an accurate picture of what is happening to a patient. They also help caregivers arrive at a diagnosis and the appropriate treatment regimen.

Diagnostic tests can be invasive and/or non-invasive. Nurses should be able to do non-invasive diagnostic tests such as blood glucose monitoring and electrocardiogram. Before starting any test, it is necessary to confirm the doctor's order for the tests and that the right patient is getting the proper test.

The testing kits and equipment should be prepared and readily available before starting any diagnostic test. The nurse should do a brief introduction of the whole process. The patient must give consent to the test before proceeding. Proper handwashing before and after the test is essential to keep the process aseptic. Afterward, the nurse should dispose of used equipment appropriately.

Blood glucose monitoring is a non-invasive procedure. The nurse should use the right strip and meter. The nurse cleans the patient's finger with an alcohol swab to disinfect it. A rapid needle prick is done on the side of the finger using a lancet. The nurse turns the finger downward to allow the blood to flow. Then the nurse wipes off the first drop of blood with a sterile gauze and collects the next drops of blood on the strip. To stop the blood, the nurse applies pressure over the puncture site with sterile gauze until the blood stops flowing. The meter then reads the blood glucose level from the strip. Blood glucose level is essential in managing patients with diabetes.

Similarly, the electrocardiogram (ECG) is a noninvasive diagnostic test that traces the heart's electrical activities. In the ECG, leads are placed on the exposed chest, hands, and legs. The activities of the heart are read on an electrocardiograph.

Laboratory Values

Some diagnostic tests require comparing the patient's test values to the standard laboratory or reference value. Laboratory tests are necessary to assess the levels of chemicals, hormones, enzymes, waste products, and even markers in various body fluids and specimens.

Specimens collected for laboratory testing include blood, urine, feces, semen, saliva, and other body tissues. Collection of these samples requires skill, practice, and proper knowledge. These tests can frighten some patients, especially pediatric patients who might fear needles and syringes. The nurse should explain the process to the patient as with any other test and obtain consent.

Blood samples can be collected in three ways: arterial sampling, venipuncture sampling, and finger prick sampling. Venipuncture is the most common way to collect blood from an adult patient. The nurse collects blood from a superficial vein in the upper limb where the vein is easily accessible. The skin is cleaned with an alcohol swab, and the arm is tied with a tourniquet to make the veins more visible. A cannula is introduced into the vein slowly. The blood is then collected into a bottle.

Venipuncture is the process of collecting blood from veins. It is a relatively safe procedure but can also have complications for both the patient and the nurse. The patient is at risk of infection from a contaminated cannula and may develop a hematoma. There's also the risk of injury to the skin, excessive bleeding, and delayed wound healing. The nurse is mainly at risk of needle pricks. Needle pricks predispose nurses to contract infections such as hepatitis B and retroviral disease. Therefore, blood sampling must be done carefully and systematically.

Urine is another sample that is collected for laboratory testing. Urine is routinely collected for urinary tract infections, sexually transmitted infections, and renal diseases. Proteins, blood cells, glucose, and other chemicals are assayed in the urine. A routine urine sample is collected in a container. The patient voids some urine into the container. The container is shut tightly, labeled properly, and taken to the laboratory for testing. Urine collection can be performed as a one-time random sample or as a 24-hour collection, depending on the specific requirements of the testing.

The nurse should compare standard reference values with the samples collected from the patient. The results can either confirm or rule out a differential diagnosis.

Recognize potential for alteration in body systems.

A nurse is expected to recognize patients with potential risks of complications and adverse disease conditions.

Due to various treatment procedures, patients have a risk of alteration in their body systems. For instance, some patients have a chance of aspiration. The entry of secretions, fluids, and solids into the tracheobronchial tree is a significant risk to specific patients. Patients with nasogastric feeding tubes are at risk of aspiration of oropharyngeal or gastrointestinal secretions. Patients with an impaired gag or cough reflex find it challenging to expel contaminants in the airway, so these stray into the lungs and block the airway. Sedated patients are also at risk of aspiration.

Other patients have a risk of potential skin breakdown. Patients who are malnourished and don't eat a balanced diet have a chance of skin breakdown because the nutrients to strengthen the connective skin tissues are absent. Malnourished patients, especially in the pediatric population, have weak immune systems and are prone to infections.

Also, patients with impaired tissue perfusion and blood circulation have a potential risk of skin breakdown because not enough blood goes to the body tissues and skin. There's also a higher chance of loss of skin tone.

Other patients are predisposed to impaired or insufficient vascular perfusion. A patient who has had a traumatic injury is at risk of impaired tissue perfusion with blood. A patient who doesn't breathe well and is hyperventilating does not have enough oxygen in the blood to perfuse the tissues. Thus, the patient is at risk of tissue hypoperfusion. This hypoperfusion can lead to shock, organ damage, and even death.

Patients exposed to cigarette smoke are at risk of lung, esophageal, and oral cancers. Patients with a family history of cancer are also at risk. Patients whose occupation exposes them to ultraviolet radiation are predisposed to skin cancers.

This knowledge will help the nurse identify patients at risk of various diseases quickly. After identifying these patients, it's important to educate them on how to avoid complications and avoid developing other diseases that they are at risk for.

Recognize potential for complications from certain diagnostic tests, treatments, or procedures.

Invasive diagnostic tests are prone to complications. For instance, invasive procedures are prone to infections and bleeding. Also, diseases such as leukemia and esophageal varices are prone to bleeding. The nurse must anticipate this and look for signs of infection or bleeding in patients.

Severe bleeding can present with features such as hypotension, tachycardia, hyperventilation, and abnormal breathing patterns because of acidosis in the blood. These signs and symptoms should be quickly noted, and treatment should follow immediately. The treatment focuses on restoring the fluids and blood cells lost in the blood. Transfusion of fluids such as ringer's lactate, blood cells, or whole blood is an option.

Infections can present with a persistent fever that may be resistant to antipyretics and tepid sponging. A blood culture may be required to detect the presence of microorganisms. The patient may also intake broad-spectrum antibiotics initially. Asepsis should be practiced to reduce the risk of infections in any procedure.

Proper positioning of patients is crucial in treating and preventing complications. A patient who has lost a lot of blood should be placed in a Trendelenburg position to facilitate blood flow to the brain. The head of the bed should also be elevated when the patient has a feeding tube.

Insert, maintain, or remove a nasal or oral gastrointestinal tube.

To insert a nasogastric tube, first, explain to the patient what you're about to do, maintain an aseptic technique, and take informed consent. Place the patient in a high Fowler position with nares adequately inspected. Select the best nares and measure the nasogastric from the nose to the tip of the xiphoid bone. Apply a topical or local anesthetic to the tube tip and put it into the nose. Flex the patient's neck slightly (into a chin-to-chest position) for proper insertion and to avoid injury to the nasopharynx. Secure the tube with a tape and a pin that attaches the tube to the patient's clothes. Connect it to a suction tube if necessary.

Removal of the tube is quite simple. Remove the pins and the tape that held the tubes in place. Ask the patient to take a deep breath and gently remove the tube. The maintenance of the nasogastric tube includes daily care. Document the drainage of the tube, the color, and the contents.

Insert, maintain, or remove a peripheral intravenous line.

This is discussed earlier in the book.

Insert, maintain, and remove a urinary catheter.

A urinary catheter is used to void urine and drain the bladder. Urinary catheters come in different sizes and differ for children and adults. Insertion of a catheter is a sterile procedure that should be done aseptically.

Place the patient in a supine position in a private room. Expose the patient's thighs and pelvic region. The patient should separate his or her thighs to give access to the perineal area. Cover the perineal area with a sterile drape. Lubricate the catheter tip and clean the urethral meatus with an antiseptic.

Insert the catheter into the urethral meatus and advance it above the point where the urine is seen in the catheter. Inflate the balloon on the catheter to secure it in the bladder. Then connect the catheter to the urine bag and attach it to the patient's leg.

In maintaining the catheter, the nurse must take proper care to maintain the aseptic nature of the bag and the tubes. The urine bag should be below the abdomen and must be emptied regularly.

Removal of the catheter must be done using aseptic techniques. Most importantly, the catheter should be removed gently, disconnected from the urine bag, and properly disposed of. The contents must be measured before the bag is emptied.

Recognize potential for complications from surgical procedures and health alterations.

Nurses must acquaint themselves with the pathophysiology of various diseases and their complications.

For instance, thrombocytopenia, a decrease in the number of platelets in the blood, can be caused by various diseases. Among them are hematological diseases of the blood, such as aplastic anemia and leukemia. HIV infection is another culprit that reduces the level of platelets in the blood. Thrombocytopenia can also be a complication of using some medications. Anticonvulsants and antibiotics reduce levels of platelets. Thrombocytopenia is mostly identified when there is difficulty arresting bleeding. It can also be asymptomatic.

Wound infection is also a complication of treatment procedures such as suturing and laceration repairs. Fever, malaise, tachycardia, swelling, and pain are all features of infections. A nurse should be on the lookout for these signs and promptly treat them. Other complications to watch for after surgery are shock and hemorrhage.

Perform system-specific assignments.

A comprehensive health assessment must be performed by a nurse when seeing a patient. A focused health assessment helps assess a specific body system.

For instance, assessing the neurological system requires assessing the cranial nerves, level of consciousness, muscle tone, and mental status. A patient's level of consciousness is determined by their orientation to time, place, and person. Patients aren't fully conscious if they don't know the time of the day, are confused about the date, or don't know where they are.

Muscle strength and tone are assessed on both the right and left of the body. Weak muscles may mean a defect in the central nervous system. They may also mean a peripheral problem. The nurse can assess the muscles and score them from 0 to 5. The muscles score zero if there's no visible contraction and score five if there's a full contraction against high resistance levels.

The 12 cranial nerves are assessed systematically. For example, the olfactory nerve is evaluated for its ability to smell. In contrast, the facial nerve is assessed for the ability to feel sensory impulses of the face and move the muscles of the face to make facial expressions.

As part of systemic-specific assignments, the glycemic level can be assessed through various signs and symptoms. Hypoglycemia symptoms include lethargy, sweating, clumsiness, loss of consciousness, coma, and even death. Hyperglycemia symptoms include polydipsia, urinary frequency, blurred vision, dehydration, and fatigue.

Therapeutic Procedures

Anesthesia can be performed for therapeutic or diagnostic procedures. It prevents a client from feeling pain that would have been otherwise unbearable during a procedure. Anesthesia can be regional, local, or general. Regional anesthesia is usually preferable to general anesthesia because of the side effects and risks of general anesthesia.

Regional anesthesia includes spinal anesthesia, where an anesthetic is injected into the subarachnoid space. The sites for administration are typically between the L3/L4 or L4/L5 vertebrae. Epidural anesthesia is a form of regional anesthesia where an anesthetic is injected into the epidural space above the dura mater.

General anesthesia makes the client completely unconscious. The patient is intubated and placed on mechanical ventilation throughout the procedure. The process is laborious and requires continuous monitoring. It is essential to monitor the amount of anesthetic given as it can have dangerous side effects.

Surgical procedures are sometimes the only form of therapy that can address a condition, such as tumors.

A nurse should explain each procedure's benefits, risks, and side effects to the patient. Every patient has the right to reject a treatment.

A nurse must take informed consent before starting a treatment procedure.

Physiological Adaptation

Physiological adaptation in nursing refers to the care of patients with acute, chronic, or life-threatening conditions. Physiological adaptation is multidisciplinary, but nurses are at the center of the action.

Monitor alterations in the body system.

The body has a system of checks and balances by which it regulates its functions. It also has repair mechanisms for damaged tissues and breakdown. The body can be affected by both external and internal insults. Internal insults are caused by internal malfunctions or disease processes. These can result in accumulated waste products, increased blood pressure, and even electrolyte imbalances. External insults can be foreign bodies or microorganisms introduced into the body.

External insults can result in internal injury. A traumatic injury with loss of blood can result in a lot of internal malfunctions with attendant consequences such as shock, infection, loss of consciousness, and death.

The body has various mechanisms in place to take care of these alterations. However, these mechanisms can fail sometimes.

For instance, in hypertension, the heart continues to enlarge, and hypertrophy occurs to compensate for the increased blood pressure. If this is not checked and corrected, hypertrophy can eventually lead to heart failure.

People have different pain thresholds. One patient may rate his or her level of pain 5/10 or moderate. Another may rate the same level of pain 9/10 or extreme. Both patients must be treated according to their requirements.

The presence of a robust support system is one helpful way of overcoming stress. For example, a patient in her fifties who is recently diagnosed with cervical cancer will need the support of her family members. Other coping mechanisms are humor, exercise, and a change in perception about current disease conditions.

Implement and monitor phototherapy.

Phototherapy treats neonatal hyperbilirubinemia and jaundice in both preterm and full-term infants. Bilirubin is a waste product produced from the breakdown of red blood cells. Accumulation of excess bilirubin is deposited in the skin, eyes, brain, and other internal organs.

Phototherapy uses a special type of blue light that breaks down the excess bilirubin. The light is applied directly to the infant's body. To prevent eye damage, the eyes are covered with protective patches. This method has been used for many years, but newer methods are also available. Newer methods are now available to treat neonatal jaundice.

A bilirubin blanket is another method of treating neonatal jaundice. The complications associated with the old method of phototherapy, such as hypothermia, rashes, bronzing and retinal damage, can now be entirely avoided. The bilirubin blanket uses light with filtered-out infrared and ultraviolet light. This blanket can be used for 24 hours. It can also be used at home outside the hospital setting.

The nurse must monitor the phototherapy treatment to see if it is effective. Check the infant's skin color to see if the bilirubin level increases or decreases. Also, check the stool color because the end products of bilirubin are a component of the feces. Last, regularly check the laboratory levels of bilirubin.

Assist with invasive procedures.

Physicians and licensed practitioners do most invasive procedures, but nurses can assist them. Some invasive procedures include central venous line, needle biopsy, spinal tap, and intubation.

Just like any procedure, the patient must give informed consent. Explain the procedure thoroughly to the patient. Ensure a sterile environment and employ aseptic techniques.

For example, before intubating a patient for mechanical ventilation, first monitor the vital signs such as blood pressure and pulse rate. Ensure the availability of suction equipment, airway supplies, and intravenous supplies. An electrocardiogram (ECG) is not specifically tied to the intubation process, but monitoring the heart rhythm is necessary during critical care interventions.

There are two types of needle biopsy: fine needle aspiration and core needle. For a needle biopsy, position the patient appropriately to expose the area of interest. Clean the area with an antiseptic and cover it with a sterile drape. Inject a local anesthetic to numb the area for a few minutes. Slowly insert the needle and obtain the specimen. Send the specimen to the laboratory for examination and cover the biopsy site with a sterile dressing.

Monitor and care for patients on a ventilator.

Ventilators push a combination of air and oxygen into the airways using pressure. This positive pressure keeps the alveoli open and facilitates gaseous exchange in the blood that flows through the pulmonary capillaries adjacent to the alveoli. Ventilators increase the oxygen saturation of a patient and lung capacity. They also decrease the breathing workload on the patient.

Nurses must be aware of the complications of using ventilators. For instance, the alveoli can overdistend due to increased air pressure from the ventilator. This overdistension can lead to pneumothorax and increased breathing work in the patient.

Oxygen toxicity is another complication. There is a tendency for the blood to be oversaturated with oxygen. Regular monitoring of the oxygen saturation level and level of carbon dioxide on the arterial blood gas machine is a way of preventing oxygen toxicity.

Infections are another possibility. Bacteria and microbes can hide in the inner lining of ventilator tubes and cause infections in patients. Pneumonia is a common disease acquired by patients on ventilators. Basic aseptic techniques such as handwashing can prevent the transfer of bacteria to patients.

Perform suctioning.

Suctioning is the mechanical aspiration of pulmonary secretions from the airways. When suctioning, the airways, including the nose, nasopharyngeal, tracheal, and other artificial airways must always be kept patent.

Administer oxygen before suctioning to pre-oxygenate the patient and prevent hypoxia during the procedure. Wear a sterile glove, and lubricate the tip of the suction catheter. Slowly advance the catheter into the patient's airways to remove secretions. This process can be repeated until the airways are clear.

Perform wound care and dressing change.

Wounds can be open or closed. Closed wounds are usually due to blunt trauma and can result in internal bleeding and closed fractures. Wounds usually require some level of dressing and care. Open wounds can be abrasions, punctures, lacerations, gunshot wounds, or surgical wounds.

Wound care and dressing change is an aseptic procedure. Clean the wound first with normal saline. If needed, antiseptic solutions such as povidone-iodine can be used, but methylated spirits are not commonly used for wound cleaning due to their potential for irritation. Clean the wound from inside to outside, from the less contaminated area to the most contaminated area. Then use a gauze to remove any debris and pus.

Inspect the wound area regularly. Examine the color, size, presence of pus, surrounding structures and odor of the pus. The drainages of the wound can be bloody, serous, serosanguinous, or purulent. After cleaning, use a new gauze or bandage plaster to dress the wound.

The frequency of dressing depends on factors such as the nature of the wound, the location, how much discharge is being produced, infections, and the preference of the physician.

Perform postoperative care.

Postoperative care is given to a patient after a surgical procedure. It is a critical part of the recovery process of any patient.

Monitor the patient after surgery. Examine the vital signs first. Measure the pulse rate and blood pressure. Examine the respiratory system. Patients just recovering from general anesthesia in surgery are at a risk of aspiration and laryngospasms. They may also feel some lightheadedness and drowsiness, which will eventually wear off. You can reassure the patients.

Patients that have had spinal anesthesia should remain flat or avoid significant elevation of the head for several hours after the procedure to prevent postdural puncture headaches. Epidural anesthesia usually does not carry the same recommendation.

Always ensure that the postoperative order is adequately documented and followed. Make any clarifications before commencing care.

Monitor a patient with a cast for pain and limb alignment. Also, monitor the patient's limb pulses and vital signs.

Provide pulmonary hygiene.

Pulmonary hygiene consists of techniques to clear the airways. The airway structures should be patent at all times so that air can flow in and out freely. Simple hygiene techniques include coughing, deep breathing, and postural drainage. Advanced techniques include percussion and vibrations.

Coughing and deep breathing are simple techniques that can be done by asking the patient to take a deep breath through the nose and exhale through the mouth. This is done three times, followed by coughing. This process can be repeated as much as possible to clear the airways.

Postural drainage involves placing the patient in various positions to promote the drainage of mucus from different parts of the lungs. For example, having the patient lie on one side can help drain the lower lobes of the lungs. The specific positions and angles depend on which part of the lung is targeted for drainage. The patient can lay supine with the head of the bed elevated to 45 degrees to drain the anterior apical segment of the upper lobes of the lungs.

Percussion is an advanced technique where the practitioner uses a cupped hand to tap over different areas of the chest to help loosen mucus. The patient is prone and the bed is elevated to a 45-degree position. Percussion is usually done with postural drainage.

Postural drainage is very useful in patients with conditions that produce excessive secretions, such as COPD or bronchiectasis.

Provide ostomy care and education.

Ostomies are surgical operations that can be done to divert the bowels (e.g., colostomy, ileostomy). Tracheostomies are performed to create an opening in the neck to access the trachea. Ostomy care and education involves informing the patient about the ostomy, its purpose, the risks of the surgery, and care after the surgery. All these responsibilities lie in the hands of a nurse.

Examine the surgical wound site as part of care for ostomies. Maintain the tubes' patency and change them as necessary. For tracheostomies, monitor the respiratory secretion inputs and outputs. Ensure that the tubes are patent and changed at the right time.

Do not neglect other routine care while taking care of the surgery site. These include vital sign monitoring and fluid input/output.

Manage the care of clients receiving peritoneal dialysis.

Dialysis replaces the function of the kidneys. This machine clears waste products from the body and balances the pH of the blood. As a result of kidney failure, waste products accumulate in the body, which is dangerous to the patient. There are two types of dialysis: hemodialysis and peritoneal dialysis.

Hemodialysis is a form of dialysis via an AV fistula, AV graft, or a central vascular line. An arteriovenous fistula or graft is created in the patient's arm to facilitate hemodialysis. The arteriovenous fistula is preferred over the graft because it has a lower risk of complications (i.e., infections). During hemodialysis, you can monitor the input and output of the patient. You can also administer any ordered anticoagulants. Record the patient's vitals, including blood pressure, pulse rate, and oxygen saturation.

Peritoneal dialysis is done by passing a catheter into the peritoneal space. This option is often chosen for patients who prefer more flexibility in their treatment schedule, those who may not tolerate hemodialysis well, or those with limited vascular access. Patients with poor venous access can get peritoneal dialysis. Measure and monitor the input and output of the patient. Also, record the color of the fluid drained out of the patient. Monitor for complications of dialysis treatment (for example, peritonitis and infections from the tubes harboring bacteria).

Fluid and Electrolyte Balance

Fluids and electrolytes are significant components of the body's internal environment. Electrolytes play a key role in maintaining the osmotic balance between the extracellular and intracellular compartments. Fluids are responsible for the function of the heart muscles and major organs of the body. These electrolytes must be monitored regularly.

Identify signs and symptoms of client fluid and/or electrolyte imbalance.

Some significant electrolytes in the body include sodium, potassium, calcium, magnesium, and chloride.

Potassium

Potassium is the most abundant intracellular electrolyte. Potassium is primarily responsible for muscle contractions and the normal functioning of the nervous system. Potassium can be high or low in the body, indicating hyperkalemia or hypokalemia.

Hyperkalemia is an elevation of the potassium levels in the blood above the expected standard value. Features of hyperkalemia include muscle paralysis, generalized body weakness, nausea, and cardiac arrhythmias. These signs are not exclusive to hyperkalemia, but hyperkalemia must be at the top of the list of possible causes. Hyperkalemia can be treated with dialysis and potassium-lowering drugs.

Hypokalemia is a reduction of the potassium levels in the blood below the normal range. Hypokalemia can be a result of diarrhea, vomiting, and diaphoresis. Hypokalemia is characterized by muscle weakness, tingling, numbness, constipation, and even cardiac arrest. Treatment is supplemental potassium.

Sodium

Sodium is responsible for the fluid balance between the extracellular and intracellular compartments of the body. Sodium also keeps the nervous system active and helps in muscle contractions. Sodium levels can be high or low in the plasma.

Hypernatremia is an elevation of the body's sodium level. Hypernatremia can arise from several illnesses and conditions such as diabetes insipidus, diarrhea, vomiting, and Cushing's syndrome. Features of hypernatremia include thirst, agitation, restlessness, and confusion. Identifying the underlying cause of hypernatremia and limiting dietary intake of sodium is critical to treating the condition.

Hyponatremia is a reduction in the sodium level in the body below the usual standard. Thyroid gland diseases, renal failure, and diuretic medications can cause hyponatremia. The condition is characterized by confusion, vomiting, nausea, headaches, and muscle weakness. Hyponatremia is treated by identifying the underlying conditions causing such. Fluid restriction and intravenous sodium are other options for treating hyponatremia.

Fluid imbalances

Hypervolemia is an increase in fluid volume in the blood. Hypervolemia is caused by increased sodium and fluid overload from the intravenous fluid infusion. The clinical features of hypervolemia are hypertension, dyspnea, shortness of breath, and peripheral edema in the feet and hands. Treatment includes sodium and fluid restrictions and treating any underlying conditions causing hypervolemia.

Hypovolemia is a reduction in the fluid in the blood. Hypovolemia may occur as a result of bleeding, vomiting, and diarrhea. This deficit in blood fluids can cause shock, reduced cardiac output, coma, and even death. Resuscitation is the first line of treatment. Infusion of intravenous fluids such as Ringer's lactate can help restore the blood volume.

Hemodynamics

Hemodynamics is the study of how blood flows through the blood vessels. It studies the factors responsible for free flow. It also studies the turbulent flow of blood in blood vessels.

Monitor and maintain arterial lines.

Arterial lines can be placed in various arteries such as the femoral, brachial, and radial arteries. These lines are inserted through a surgical procedure to monitor the patient's blood pressure. Arterial lines can also be used to obtain frequent blood samples. Nurses should know the complications, such as infections, trauma, hematomas, and scar tissue formation.

Arterial lines are used for continuous blood pressure monitoring and frequent blood sampling. Monitor the hemodynamic status of patients with arterial lines. Also, anticipate complications and manage them accordingly.

Manage the care of patients with telemetry.

Telemetry is the continuous monitoring and recording of ECG strips. It is mostly done by a telemetry technician, but nurses can also monitor telemetry. When there is a problem with the patient's ECG, the nurse has to interpret the ECG and decide on the next course of action.

Manage the care of a patient with a pacing device.

To care for a patient with a pacing device, first educate the patient about the reason for the pacemaker. The nurse should be aware of the complications of having a pacemaker. Complications of having a pacing device include pneumothorax, hemothorax, perforation of the pacemaker lead, and cardiac tamponade. These complications are identified by shortness of breath, chest pain, and low blood pressure.

Monitor the ECG for the failure of the pacemaker. Assess the insertion site of the pacemaker for bleeding and infections. Advise the patient to limit arm movement and monitor for complications after pacemaker insertion. The decision to give or withhold medications like heparin or aspirin will depend on the patient's medical condition and the physician's orders.

Illness Management

Illness management begins with educating the patient about acute and chronic conditions. The education of patients includes information about the pathophysiology of the disease condition. The nurse should be able to explain how the disease process began. Tell the patient about the risk factors predisposing to the diseases. Explain the signs and symptoms of the disease to the patient so they can be reported to the doctor if present.

Also, explain the signs and symptoms of chronic diseases to the patient and which ones can be managed or treated. Tell them about the treatment procedures and the financial cost of each treatment. Teach patients about home care strategies for their illnesses. Patients should receive the follow-up schedule as part of the treatment plan.

Patients with impaired ventilation or oxygenation should be assessed with pulmonary function tests such as pulse oximetry, spirometry, lung compliance, and forced vital capacity. Manage these patients by regularly monitoring the results of these tests.

Test 1 Questions

(1) A woman presents at the hospital in the second stage of labor. What should a nurse expect at this stage?

(A) Braxton-Hicks contraction.

(B) 2 cm cervical dilatation.

(C) Delivery of the fetus.

(D) 6 cm cervical dilatation.

(2) A patient presents with pentazocine addiction. The nurse decides to call in a psychologist, a psychotherapist, and a physician. What has the nurse demonstrated?

(A) Crisis intervention.

(B) Recognition of appropriate resources for referral needs.

(C) Client assessment.

(D) B and C.

(3) A nurse working in the emergency room has a very busy afternoon. She has four patients who need attention: a teenager with an adverse reaction (fever and shivering) from an ongoing blood transfusion; a middle-aged man with pain from osteoarthritis in his right knee; a 25-year-old man involved in an auto crash who has lost a lot of blood; and an elderly woman in for her weekly chemotherapy. In what order should the nurse attend to the patients?

(A) Teenager, middle-aged man, elderly woman, young man.

(B) Middle-aged man, elderly woman, young man, teenager.

(C) Young man, middle-aged man, teenager, elderly woman.

(D) Teenager, young man, middle-aged man, elderly woman.

(4) Your friend's brother, Joe, calls you asking for information about one of his friends on your ward who was involved in an accident. He is aware there is a fracture but wants to know if any of his friend's organs were affected. What is your most appropriate response?

(A) "It was just his right leg."

(B) "Joe, please get off my phone. Never ask me about patient issues."

(C) "I am sorry, Joe. I can't give you that information."

(D) "Please ask your friend if he wants me to tell you."

(5) The physician on call the previous shift forgot to document a medication to be given at 0700 hrs. He calls to ask you to give it. What do you say?

(A) “I cannot give the medication because you did not document it.”

(B) “I cannot give the medication because you did not document it. I suggest you ask another physician to come document it.”

(C) “Please don’t tell me to do this again; it is against the law.”

(D) “I cannot give the medication because you did not document it. Verbal orders are recognized only during emergencies. I suggest you ask another physician to come document it.”

(6) Mr. Alex has always believed that he can control his fate. He has been diagnosed with cancer but still believes he must do all he can to live healthily. Mr. Alex can be said to have __________.

(A) Internal locus.

(B) External locus.

(C) Experiential readiness.

(D) Mental readiness.

(7) A mother complains about her six-year-old, who has begun to challenge her authority at home. After reassuring her that this comes with age, what should the nurse counsel her to help her child avoid?

(A) Smoking.

(B) Unsupervised swimming.

(C) Falls.

(D) All of the above.

(8) One of your junior nursing staff members refused to allow a patient to look through his medical records. What should you do as an RN?

(A) Apologize to the patient and allow him to view his records.

(B) Support your staff.

(C) Educate your staff on HIPAA.

(D) All of the above.

(9) A patient presents with a persistent fever that is resistant to antipyretics. The patient might urgently need all the following except a/an __________.

(A) CBC.

(B) Blood culture.

(C) EUCR.

(D) CT scan.

(10) A patient is observed to experience cardiac arrhythmias. What investigation should be ordered immediately and why?

(A) CBC, infection.

(B) Blood culture, infection.

(C) Peripheral blood film, leukemia.

(D) EUCR, hyperkalemia.

(11) An 80-year-old woman is a known patient with diabetes mellitus and has been in treatment for over 30 years. She is admitted for a routine check-up. Which of the following basic assessments is most important in this patient?

(A) Mobility assessment.

(B) Hearing assessment.

(C) Speech assessment.

(D) Visual assessment.

(12) A 65-year-old man was admitted to the ER complaining of an inability to pass stool for the past week. Previous digital rectal examination findings revealed a full rectum with hardened stool. As the nurse on duty, what is your most likely assessment?

(A) Constipation.

(B) Fecal impaction.

(C) Intestinal obstruction.

(D) Volvulus.

(13) During a mobility assessment of a patient admitted for thoracic spine transection, which of these statements is true?

(A) Mobility issues are acquired from predisposing factors.

(B) Muscle contraction as a parameter for mobility assessment is scored on a scale of 0 to 6.

(C) Mobility issues can affect other systems aside from the musculoskeletal system.

(D) Mobility issues are usually unifactorial.

(14) A 50-year-old woman being managed for advanced breast cancer complains of pain. Which of the following is true about pain management and evaluation?

(A) Acute pain is usually described based on the severity of the pain.

(B) Pharmacological treatment is always indicated in pain management.

(C) Pain is usually a complication of treatment in oncology cases.

(D) Nonpharmacological comfort interventions can be effective in the management of pain.

(15) A patient was placed on amitriptyline and lorazepam to manage major depression. The patient is complaining of excessive somnolence. What is the next best course of action?

(A) Increase the dosage of the medication.

(B) Stop the medication immediately.

(C) Document for a possible revision of medications and reduction of dosage.

(D) Dissuade the patient's fears and continue the current medication at the present dosage.

(16) An unconscious patient was admitted with a cervical and thoracic spine fracture following an RTA. What is the most appropriate method to prevent bed sores in this patient?

(A) Regular turning in bed.

(B) Use of a waterbed.

(C) Adequate rehydration.

(D) Regular application of zinc oxide cream.

(17) A patient who injected a toxic substance that is primarily eliminated by the kidneys is brought to the ER. Which of the following is an ineffective method to enhance renal elimination?

(A) Increased intravenous fluid intake.

(B) Administration of diuretics.

(C) Ensured adequate blood flow and perfusion.

(D) Suprapubic (bladder) massage.

(18) A patient was admitted and managed for constipation. What is not an appropriate part of the evaluation and care of the patient?

(A) Increased intravenous fluid intake.

(B) Assessment of dietary intake.

(C) Assessment of bowel habits.

(D) Possible enema if indicated.

(19) A 12-year-old child who is being managed for sepsis runs a fever with a temperature of 39.1 °C. What action is not appropriate?

(A) Administer antipyretics.

(B) Expose the child adequately and use tepid sponging.

(C) Increase fluid intake.

(D) Encourage ambulation.

(20) A patient is being treated for traumatic brain injury following a road traffic accident. The patient is observed to be confused. What is an inappropriate line of care for this patient?

(A) Sedate the patient.

(B) Ensure the bed railings are up.

(C) Lightly restrain the patient in bed.

(D) Adequately counsel the relatives.

(21) A 35-year-old woman is being evaluated for cholecystitis. She is found to be morbidly obese and has been previously diagnosed with binge eating. Which counsel is inappropriate?

(A) Avoidance/reduction of fatty meal intake and fast foods.

(B) Weight reduction.

(C) Frequent small meals.

(D) Regular fasting.

(22) An unconscious patient is being managed in the intensive care unit by the nurse on duty. What is an inappropriate way to feed this patient?

(A) Commence total parenteral nutrition where available.

(B) Spoon-feed the patient while propped up in bed.

(C) Ensure glucose-containing intravenous fluids are given.

(D) Pass an orogastric tube to feed with a blended diet.

(23) A seven-month-old infant is brought to the pediatric outpatient clinic on account of poor weight gain following weaning off breast milk. What is an inappropriate question to ask when evaluating this patient?

(A) Weaning diet.

(B) History of maternal illness in pregnancy.

(C) Birth and current weight of the child.

(D) Appetite and dietary habit.

(24) A 68-year-old woman has left hip hemiarthroplasty for an acetabular fracture. Which mobility assistive device is best to use with this patient?

(A) Zimmer's walking frame.

(B) Elbow crutches.

(C) Walking cane.

(D) Wheelchair.

(25) Matt has smoked for 17 years. His doctor has confirmed some lung changes that are looking carcinogenic, but Matt still smokes. What is the term for this?

(A) Dependence.

(B) Addiction.

(C) Withdrawal symptoms.

(D) Substance abuse.

(26) A patient presents to the ER complaining of an inability to sleep. On examination, you find he has needle marks on his upper limbs. He is also moving slowly and has remarkably poor hygiene. What should your next steps be?

(A) Call the police.

(B) Evaluate the patient using CAGE-AID.

(C) Refer the patient.

(D) Prescribe medications for his symptoms.

(27) A patient diagnosed with stage IV breast cancer has been unable to eat since she received the news. She used to be lively but has now become very depressed. Her family members are concerned. You notice she is looking dehydrated and weak. What can you do to help?

(A) Set up infusions.

(B) Refer the patient to a psychologist.

(C) Counsel the relatives.

(D) All of the above.

(28) Chris lost his father two days ago, but he has repeatedly asked him to come back. He says that his dad just took one of his long evening walks and will soon come back home. What stage of the Kübler-Ross model is this?

(A) Denial.

(B) Depression.

(C) Bargaining.

(D) Acceptance.

(29) A woman presents with a very low PCV. On taking her history, you find she does not believe in or want a blood transfusion. What is your next course of action?

(A) Try to convince her.

(B) Document her stance and seek alternatives.

(C) Explain the risks associated with her decision.

(D) B and C.

(30) A patient with severe anemia is being transfused, and 30 minutes later, he is noticed to be febrile and tachycardic. What will your next line of action be?

(A) Stop the transfusion and inform the doctor.

(B) Continue the transfusion, give corticosteroids and antihistamines, and inform the doctor.

(C) Stop the transfusion, give normal saline, and inform the doctor.

(D) Continue the transfusion, give normal saline, antihistamines and corticosteroids, and inform the doctor.

(31) A patient with blood type O receives type B blood. What type of reaction will occur?

(A) Allergic blood reaction.

(B) Delayed hypersensitivity reaction.

(C) Hemolytic transfusion reaction.

(D) None, the blood types are compatible.

(32) A patient had peripheral venous access one day ago, and during the administration of vancomycin, the patient complained of intense pain and heat in the arm. Pain subsided afterward, and upon administration of sterile injection water, there was no pain. What is the nurse's next line of action?

(A) Remove IV access to prevent infection.

(B) Reassure the patient and inform the doctor.

(C) Do nothing.

(D) None of the above.

(33) A two-year-old boy was brought into the children's emergency department with a history of seven episodes of vomiting and nine episodes of the passage of loose stool over the past 24 hours, with signs of severe dehydration. What is the most appropriate route for resuscitation in this patient?

(A) Oral route.

(B) Intramuscular route.

(C) Intravenous route.

(D) Transdermal route.

(34) You are admitting an elderly patient named Mr. Johnson who hands you a document titled "Advance Directives" which states his preferences for medical care should he become unable to make decisions himself. This document is known as what?

(A) A document provided in advance of a medical condition.

(B) A document given when the patient is in a coma.

(C) Legal documentation outlining how a patient should be managed at all times.

(D) Legal documentation defining how patients should be handled if they are unable to communicate.

(35) As a nurse, Mrs. Smith informs you that she has prepared advanced directives. What is your responsibility regarding these directives?

(A) Document them in Mrs. Smith's records.

(B) Inform other healthcare personnel who need to be aware of the directives.

(C) Ensure that the directives are followed should the need arise.

(D) All of the above.

(36) As a head nurse, you decide on tasks that you can delegate to a nursing assistant. What kind of tasks are usually safe to delegate?

(A) Set routine tasks.

(B) Tasks that require a lower level of professional judgment.

(C) Care needs for patients in stable condition.

(D) Tasks that require quick judgment calls.

(37) You are training a new nurse on delegation. When you discuss the five rights of delegation, which of the following options is correct?

(A) Right person, task, perception, circumstance, supervision.

(B) Right person, task, circumstance, direction, supervision.

(C) Right person, task, skill, direction, supervision.

(D) Right person, task, equipment, remuneration, supervision.

(38) Your hospital has a healthcare reimbursement system where payments are received based on the cost of care provided. What is this system called?

(A) Prospective reimbursement.

(B) Retrogressive reimbursement.

(C) Progressive reimbursement.

(D) Retrospective reimbursement.

(39) You are working with a team to create a healthcare plan for a patient named Jane. What essential aspect should be considered when developing Jane's plan?

(A) Individualization.

(B) Movement.

(C) Evaluation.

(D) All of the above.

(40) According to the Patient's Bill of Rights, what choices do patients have when it comes to their healthcare?

(A) They can select their healthcare provider.

(B) They can reject healthcare plans that they do not want.

(C) They can choose the type of healthcare plan that they want.

(D) All of the above.

(41) You are advocating for a patient's needs with your healthcare team. What action is not typically part of your role as an advocate?

(A) Update other nursing staff about patient advocacy.

(B) Document the needs of the patient.

(C) Communicate the needs of patients orally to other nursing staff.

(D) Take on multiple roles for effectiveness.

(42) You are assisting in a resuscitation effort for a patient who has gone into cardiac arrest. What is the correct order of steps to follow in resuscitation?

(A) Airway, breathing, circulation.

(B) Breathing, airway, circulation.

(C) Circulation, breathing, airway.

(D) Circulation, airway, breathing.

(43) You are orienting a new nurse to your unit, which promotes a culture of safety. You explain that the unit operates within a blameless environment. How would you describe this type of environment to the new nurse?

(A) An environment without any faults.

(B) An environment where mistakes are not often made.

(C) An environment where errors are viewed as opportunities for learning and improvement.

(D) An environment that focuses on the individual who made the error.

(44) As a nurse manager, you are examining the statistics for your unit, such as the number of patients admitted each day and the total number of patients in the unit. What kind of measures would you use to assess these values?

(A) Core measures.

(B) Outcome measures.

(C) Quality measures.

(D) Quantity measures.

(45) As a quality improvement nurse, you're facilitating a meeting to address a recently identified issue in patient care. Which of the following steps is typically part of every performance improvement methodology?

(A) Define the problem.

(B) Perform a root cause analysis.

(C) Narrow down the issue.

(D) All of the above.

(46) A patient has just been brought into the ER with a severe head injury and is currently unstable. Which of the following healthcare professionals are best suited to manage this critical case?

(A) Licensed Practical Nurses (LPNs).

(B) Registered Nurses (RNs).

(C) Nursing assistants.

(D) All of the above.

(47) You are a nurse in a pediatric ward and have noticed signs of child abuse in one of your patients. Who among the healthcare team should be involved in this case?

(A) Physical therapists.

(B) Occupational therapists.

(C) Nutritionists.

(D) Social workers.

(48) During a staff meeting, a conflict arises between two team members. One of them begins to rationalize their actions that led to the conflict. At which stage of the conflict process does this occur?

(A) Frustration.

(B) Anger.

(C) Conceptualization.

(D) Action.

(49) You're teaching a class on conflict resolution strategies for nursing students. Which of the following groups of methods would you classify as unhealthy approaches to resolving conflicts?

(A) Avoidance, competition, mediation.

(B) Mediation, compromise, collaboration.

(C) Avoidance, accommodating without addressing issues, competition.

(D) None of the above.

(50) You're prioritizing patient care in a busy ICU. Which of the following factors should not influence your decisions when determining priorities?

(A) Pathophysiology.

(B) Acuity.

(C) Race.

(D) All of the above.

(51) You're evaluating the effectiveness of a new treatment plan implemented for a patient in your care. On what basis would you determine the success of this plan?

(A) The cost of care.

(B) The acuity of care.

(C) The patient's recovery progress.

(D) Whether the disease follows the expected pathophysiology.

(52) As a nursing professional, you encounter ethical dilemmas from time to time. What is a common feature of these ethical challenges?

(A) The ethical standards conflict with the nurse's personal beliefs.

(B) The ethical standards conflict with the patient's interests.

(C) The patient's interests align with the ethical standards.

(D) The patient has no influence in the ethical dilemma.

(53) As a nurse manager, you're conducting evaluations of your nursing staff. A new nurse asks you what the purpose of these evaluations is. How do you respond?

(A) The evaluations help nurses better fulfill their duties.

(B) The evaluations are not relevant.

(C) The evaluations only benefit those in upper management.

(D) None of the above.

(54) You're a charge nurse, and you're reviewing charting entries made by a newly hired nurse. The entry reads "08/12/20 1020 hrs. IM Diclofenac 75 mg stat given. Pain has subsided." What would be the most accurate way for this information to be recorded?

(A) 09/12/20 1020 hrs. IM Diclofenac 75 mg stat given. Pain has subsided.

(B) 09/12/20 1020 hrs. IM Diclofenac 75 mg total dose given. Patient reports pain level as 2/10.

(C) 09/12/20 1020 hrs. IV Diclofenac 75 mg given. Patient states they are feeling better.

(D) 09/12/20 1020 hrs. IM Diclofenac 75 mg STAT given. Patient reports pain level as 2/10.

(55) You have been assigned to a patient who is blind. What methods would you use to effectively communicate with this patient?

(A) Signs.

(B) Speaking.

(C) Braille.

(D) Both B and C.

(56) As a public health nurse, you're responsible for screening programs. When would you typically perform targeted screening?

(A) During a patient's routine check-up.

(B) When a patient is at high risk for a specific disease.

(C) To rule out a specific condition in a patient.

(D) Both B and C.

(57) You are conducting a health history interview with a new patient. What does NOT typically occur during a health history assessment?

(A) Ask open-ended questions.

(B) Ask closed-ended questions.

(C) Conduct an interview-style questioning.

(D) Help patients express themselves more.

(58) You are working as a nurse in a clinic that provides sexual health services. A patient comes in who admits to regularly having unprotected sex with multiple partners. How can you assist this patient?

(A) Advise abstinence.

(B) Advise the use of condoms.

(C) Counsel about the risks of having multiple sexual partners.

(D) All of the above.

(59) As a community health nurse, you visit a family where the children appear malnourished. What could you do to help prevent malnutrition in this family?

(A) Educate the parents on the importance of a balanced diet.

(B) Teach the children about what constitutes a balanced diet.

(C) Counsel the parents on various cooking techniques.

(D) Provide financial counseling to the parents.

(60) You are working as a community health nurse, and your goal is to encourage health-promoting behaviors among your patients. How would you evaluate your patients' understanding of these behaviors?

(A) Observe their actions.

(B) Ask formal and informal questions about their health behaviors.

(C) Have them complete questionnaires about their lifestyle habits.

(D) All of the above.

(61) As a pediatric nurse, you are caring for an infant patient. A medical student on rotation asks about the developmental stage the infant is likely in, according to Piaget's theory. What is your response?

(A) Neonatal stage.

(B) Sensorimotor stage.

(C) Preoperational stage.

(D) Concrete operational stage.

(62) As a geriatric nurse, you are providing care for a patient in her 50s. According to Erik Erikson's stages of psychosocial development, what might be some of the key concerns for someone in this stage, known as "generativity vs. stagnation"?

(A) Caring for children and aging parents.

(B) Finding a sense of purpose in life.

(C) Dealing with feelings of self-consciousness.

(D) Preparing for retirement.

(63) You are explaining to a nursing student the importance of considering decreased hepatic and renal function when caring for elderly patients. What is the primary significance of this consideration?

(A) It helps prevent falls.

(B) It affects how the body metabolizes prescription medications.

(C) It can lead to feelings of isolation from family.

(D) All of the above.

(64) You are working as an obstetric nurse. A pregnant patient asks you what the most accurate method is for determining her estimated due date (EDD). What do you tell her?

(A) The first day of her last menstrual period (LMP).

(B) An ultrasound scan done in the first trimester of pregnancy.

(C) The date of ovulation.

(D) The day the patient first felt nausea.

(65) As a pediatric nurse, you are instructing new parents how to care for their newborn's umbilical cord at home. What do you recommend they use to clean it?

(A) Alcohol.

(B) Normal saline.

(C) Warm water.

(D) All of the above.

(66) In the ER, a patient presents with symptoms you suspect could be an allergic reaction. What symptoms might these be?

(A) Difficulty breathing.

(B) Hypotension.

(C) A tingling sensation.

(D) All of the above.

(67) If a patient on your ward starts exhibiting signs of an allergic reaction, what is the correct immediate action to take?

(A) Discharge the patient as the treatment options available aren't compatible.

(B) Document the patient's allergic reaction for future reference.

(C) Move the patient to another room to alleviate the allergic reaction.

(D) Contact the Centers for Disease Control and Prevention (CDC).

(68) You are a nurse in a busy hospital ward, and there are four new admissions. Which patient should you consider the most prone to a fall?

(A) A patient experiencing mental instability and currently restrained.

(B) A 30-year-old patient who has been sedated and is unrestrained.

(C) An 83-year-old patient in a room with low-glare floors.

(D) A day-old baby in the Intensive Care Unit.

(69) You're working in a community health clinic, and a parent asks you when their child can stop using a car seat. According to most state laws, you inform them that children must remain in car seats until they are:

(A) 12 years old.

(B) 4'9" in height.

(C) Weigh 80 pounds.

(D) Either 4'9" or 80 pounds.

(70) You're a nurse caring for a patient with a history of seizures. To prepare for a possible seizure episode, what measure should you implement?

(A) Pad the patient's bed rails and elevating the bed for better positioning and comfort.

(B) Have oxygen and suction equipment readily available.

(C) Move the patient to a private room to promote privacy and reduce potential embarrassment.

(D) All of the above.

(71) You're admitting a new patient to the ward. To ensure proper identification and minimize errors, what procedures should you avoid?

(A) Paying special attention to patients who are at a higher risk of identification errors.

(B) Using identifiers, such as the patient's date of birth and medical record number.

(C) Using a single unique identifier along with the patient's room number for easy identification.

(D) Adding extra identifiers when there is more than one patient with the same name on the ward.

(72) As an RN, you receive a medication order for a patient that seems unusual or potentially harmful. Do you have the right to question this order?

(A) No.

(B) Yes.

(C) It depends on who wrote the order.

(D) It's subject to the rules of each individual healthcare facility.

(73) You're conducting a hospital orientation for a group of newly hired nurses. When discussing emergency codes, which of the following statements is incorrect?

(A) Code Gray is the appropriate code for communicating an infant abduction.

(B) Code Red and Code Orange are used for fire hazards and chemical spills, respectively.

(C) Code Blue is used to signal a cardiac arrest.

(D) Code Brown is used to indicate a severe weather disaster.

(74) You're conducting a manual handling training session for a group of newly hired nursing assistants. What actions should be avoided when managing patients and using common hospital equipment?

(A) Using the back muscles when lifting heavy objects.

(B) Facing the person or object to be lifted with feet close together.

(C) None of the above.

(D) All of the above.

(75) As an RN, you're about to assign assistive devices to your patients. Which of the following factors should influence your decision?

(A) The distance from the patient's home to the healthcare facility.

(B) The patient's religious or cultural affiliations.

(C) The patient's income level.

(D) The patient's height, weight, and muscular strength.

(76) You're supervising a new nursing intern who is learning about proper handling of biohazardous waste. Which of the following actions by the intern would violate general principles for handling such waste?

(A) The intern avoids reusing materials designed for single use.

(B) The intern properly cleans and disinfects non-single-use materials.

(C) The intern rigorously washes his hands before handling any biohazardous material.

(D) The intern disposes of biohazardous material in any available trash can.

(77) As part of your responsibilities on the medical-surgical unit, you regularly inspect all medical equipment. What should you be particularly vigilant for during these inspections?

(A) Loose or missing equipment parts.

(B) Frayed electrical cords.

(C) Overloaded power outlets.

(D) All of the above.

(78) As a nurse in a metropolitan hospital, you're part of the team that prepares for potential security threats. What actions should be a part of your preparedness plan?

(A) Delegation of security responsibilities to other staff members.

(B) Review of policies and procedures only in the event of a security breach.

(C) Participation in periodic training and mock drills.

(D) Employment of security experts who will manage situations when they arise.

(79) During your health education session with patients on infectious disease prevention, you explain the different ways pathogens can be transmitted. How do you describe these modes of transmission?

(A) Airborne, contact, droplet, and vector-borne.

(B) Airborne, droplet, direct, and indirect.

(C) Vector-borne, direct, indirect, and airborne.

(D) Contact, vector-borne, direct, and indirect.

(80) One of your patients is concerned about vector-borne diseases after a recent news outbreak about the West Nile virus. Which example would you give to explain a vector-borne transmission mode?

(A) Touching a contaminated surface and then touching one's mouth.

(B) Inhaling respiratory droplets from a person infected with a contagious disease.

(C) Getting bitten by a mosquito carrying the West Nile virus.

(D) Shaking hands with a person who has a cold.

(81) As part of your efforts to reduce hospital-acquired infections, you emphasize the importance of handwashing to your nursing team. When should handwashing be done?

(A) Before contact with a patient.

(B) When the hands have been soiled.

(C) After touching equipment, instruments, and other treatment materials with bare hands.

(D) All of the above.

(82) During a teaching session with a group of nursing students, you explain the importance of aseptic techniques. Which of the following definitions would you use to explain what aseptic techniques are?

(A) Measures taken to prevent the transfer of disease-causing organisms from one person or object to another.

(B) Measures taken to render microorganisms ineffective for causing infections.

(C) Precautionary measures used for all patients to prevent the spread of infection.

(D) Measures taken to prevent the spread of specific infections.

(83) An outbreak of a rare infectious disease has occurred on your unit. As the charge nurse, what is the appropriate procedure for reporting and communicating about this infectious disease?

(A) Reports should go to the patient's family members.

(B) Reports should go to the Centers for Disease Control and Prevention.

(C) Reports should go to the local hospital.

(D) Reports should go to the nursing assistant.

(84) You are a head nurse in an infectious disease department of a hospital. As part of your responsibilities, you are required to _______.

(A) Test all incoming patients for infection before they're admitted.

(B) Ensure all staff members strictly adhere to infection control measures.

(C) Plan and evaluate educational activities on safety for patients.

(D) Personally administer antibiotics to all infected patients.

(85) A patient in the psychiatric ward is displaying signs of agitation and potential harm to self and others. When selecting an appropriate restraint for this patient, you should consider the ___________.

(A) Patient's level of consciousness.

(B) Patient's mobility.

(C) Patient's age.

(D) Patient's preference.

(86) As a nursing student, you are learning about vital signs and how to measure them. Which of the following is not considered a vital sign?

(A) Blood pressure.

(B) Respiratory rate.

(C) Pulse rate.

(D) Body Mass Index (BMI).

(87) You are training a new nurse on how to take a patient's blood pressure. You explain that when using the stethoscope, you listen for _________.

(A) Korotkoff sounds.

(B) Waltz sounds.

(C) Lead sounds.

(D) Schmitz sounds.

(88) You are preparing to perform a blood draw on a patient. Before you begin, you should ___________.

(A) Confirm the doctor's order.

(B) Identify the patient.

(C) Prepare the materials.

(D) Both A and B.

(89) As an RN in a cardiology unit, you often use the ECG machine. What does this machine record?

(A) Electrical impulses of the heart.

(B) Sinus waves.

(C) Mechanical impulses of the heart.

(D) Potential energy of the heart.

(90) During your shift at the hospital, you're asked to collect a blood sample from a patient. Which of the following is not a method for blood sample collection?

(A) Arterial sampling.

(B) Venipuncture.

(C) Finger prick.

(D) None of the above.

(91) As a nurse, you're often required to perform venipunctures on patients. What's the most significant risk to you during this procedure?

(A) Injury to the skin.

(B) Excessive bleeding.

(C) Delayed wound healing.

(D) Needle prick.

(92) After drawing blood from a patient, you know it's important to prevent hematoma formation. How would you accomplish this?

(A) Ask the patient to flex the elbow after sample collection.

(B) Apply pressure on the sample collection site.

(C) Ensure the sample is only taken once.

(D) Remove the tourniquet as quickly as possible.

(93) You're working in a rehabilitation center where you care for a variety of patients with different conditions. Among the following patients under your care, who has the least risk of aspiration?

(A) An elderly patient with nasogastric (NG) tubes.

(B) A stroke survivor with an impaired gag reflex.

(C) A patient who is heavily sedated post-surgery.

(D) A conscious patient who recently underwent knee replacement surgery.

(94) You are an emergency room nurse, and a patient comes in from a car accident suffering from a traumatic injury with substantial blood loss. As you assess the patient, you realize that the greatest immediate concern is _________.

(A) Hypovolemic shock.

(B) Neurogenic shock.

(C) Hypothermia.

(D) Infection.

(95) As a home health nurse, you visit a patient who lives alone and has been having trouble preparing meals. Upon assessment, you note that malnourishment can lead to ________.

(A) Infections.

(B) A weak immune system.

(C) Skin breakdown.

(D) All of the above.

(96) You're a nurse in a medical surgical unit, and you're preparing to remove a nasogastric tube from a patient. Before removing the tube, you need to note the _______.

(A) Quantity of drainage.

(B) Color of the drainage.

(C) Content of the drainage.

(D) All of the above.

(97) You're starting an IV on a new patient in the ER. Where would you place the tourniquet?

(A) Below the selected site.

(B) At the selected site.

(C) A few inches above the selected site.

(D) None of the above.

(98) You are preparing to catheterize a patient with urinary retention. The catheter enters the bladder by passing through the _________.

(A) Urethral meatus.

(B) Urethra.

(C) A and B.

(D) None of the above.

(99) As a neuroscience nurse, you are assessing a patient's cranial nerves. When assessing the sense of smell, you're examining which cranial nerve?

(A) Ophthalmic nerve.

(B) Olfactory nerve.

(C) Trigeminal nerve.

(D) Optic nerve.

(100) A patient with diabetes comes to the clinic reporting feeling “off.” Upon assessment, you note several symptoms that suggest hypoglycemia. All the following symptoms might indicate hypoglycemia, except _________.

(A) Lethargy.

(B) Sweating.

(C) Polydipsia.

(D) Clumsiness.

(101) You are working as a surgical nurse and discussing anesthesia options with a patient scheduled for knee replacement surgery. You inform the patient that types of anesthesia include _______.

(A) Regional and general.

(B) Full and partial.

(C) Strong and weak.

(D) Upper limb block and lower limb block.

(102) You’re working as an obstetric nurse and discussing pain relief options with a laboring patient. The patient is considering receiving anesthesia above the dura mater. What kind of anesthesia would this be?

(A) Spinal.

(B) Epidural.

(C) Bier’s block.

(D) General anesthesia.

(103) As an emergency room nurse, a patient arrives with a gunshot wound. In terms of classification, a gunshot injury would be considered what type of insult?

(A) External.

(B) Internal.

(C) Internal and external.

(D) None of the above.

(104) You're explaining the results of a liver function test to a patient. The patient has elevated bilirubin levels. You explain that bilirubin is formed from the _________.

(A) Breakdown of fats.

(B) Breakdown of red blood cells (RBCs).

(C) Formation of RBCs.

(D) Breakdown of hepatocytes.

(105) As an OR nurse, you are about to assist with an invasive procedure. The initial steps before performing this procedure would include _______.

(A) Gathering materials.

(B) Obtaining informed consent.

(C) Explaining the procedure to the patient.

(D) All of the above.

(106) You are a critical care nurse attending to a patient who was recently placed on a ventilator. When explaining the purpose of the ventilator to the patient's family, you would say that ventilators are used:

(A) To increase the breathing workload of the patient.

(B) To reduce the breathing workload of the patient.

(C) For procedures that require local anesthesia.

(D) For procedures that require conscious sedation.

(107) You're working in a respiratory care unit, and a new nurse asks you to explain suctioning. You would describe suctioning as the ________.

(A) Natural aspiration of pulmonary secretions.

(B) Artificial use of air to prevent the collapse of the lungs.

(C) Artificial aspiration of pulmonary secretions.

(D) Preoxygenation of the patient before surgery.

(108) You're about to change the dressing on a patient's wound. You gather the necessary supplies, which do not include _______.

(A) Povidone.

(B) Methylated spirit.

(C) Honey.

(D) None of the above.

(109) As a post-anesthesia care unit (PACU) nurse, upon receiving a patient from surgery, the first step you should perform is _______.

(A) Take the patient's vital signs.

(B) Check the surgery site.

(C) Request postoperative orders.

(D) Request handover notes.

(110) You're providing patient education on how to maintain pulmonary hygiene at home. Simple techniques you suggest include _______.

(A) Coughing, deep breathing, and vibrations.

(B) Deep breathing, vibrations, and percussion.

(C) Vibrations and percussion.

(D) Coughing and postural drainage.

(111) As a surgical nurse, you are preparing a patient for an ostomy. In explaining the procedure to the patient, you tell them that ostomies are surgical operations done to create _______.

(A) Heart chambers.

(B) Openings from the outside to the inside.

(C) Organs.

(D) Openings from the inside to the outside.

(112) You are a nurse at a dialysis center caring for a patient undergoing peritoneal dialysis. You know that a potential complication of this procedure that you should monitor for is ___________.

(A) Peritonitis.

(B) Headaches.

(C) Vomiting.

(D) Swollen lower limbs.

(113) You're educating a patient who will soon start dialysis via an AV graft. The patient asks where this graft is typically positioned. You tell them it is usually located at the _________.

(A) Upper limb.

(B) Lower thigh.

(C) Chest.

(D) Elbow.

(114) In educating a group of nursing students about the body's electrolytes, you ask them to identify which of the following is not an electrolyte in the body.

(A) Sodium.

(B) Magnesium.

(C) Calcium.

(D) Mercury.

(115) You are reviewing lab results for a patient who has been diagnosed with hyponatremia. When considering possible causes, you understand that a common cause of this condition could be _________.

(A) Diuretics.

(B) Dialysis.

(C) Vomiting.

(D) Headaches.

(116) As a critical care nurse, you are monitoring a patient for signs of hypovolemia. You know that one severe complication of this condition that could quickly lead to death if not addressed is _________.

(A) Vomiting.

(B) Hypothermia.

(C) Shock.

(D) All of the above.

(117) During a critical care nursing lecture, you are discussing the use of blood volume expanders. The examples you provide include ___________.

(A) 50% dextrose water.

(B) 50% dextrose saline.

(C) Ringer's lactate.

(D) Mannitol.

(118) You are a telemetry nurse explaining your role to a patient. You explain that telemetry involves _________.

(A) Continuous monitoring of an EEG.

(B) Continuous monitoring and recording of an ECG.

(C) One-time measurement and recording of an ECG.

(D) None of the above.

(119) As an emergency room nurse, you are assessing a patient who has been in a car accident. The patient is presenting with shortness of breath, and the chest does not seem to rise fully on one side. You suspect that the patient may be experiencing a ________.

(A) Hemothorax.

(B) Pneumothorax.

(C) Rib fracture.

(D) Lung contusion.

(120) You are inserting an arterial line for a critically ill patient in the ICU. The purpose of this line is to _________.

(A) Monitor the patient's blood pressure.

(B) Obtain frequent blood samples.

(C) A and B.

(D) None of the above.

(121) You're a respiratory therapist working in a pulmonology clinic. A patient with chronic obstructive pulmonary disease (COPD) is scheduled for an assessment of their lung function. You are preparing to perform several tests that fall under the category of _________.

(A) Spirometry.

(B) Blood glucose.

(C) Chest X-rays.

(D) Chest CT scans.

(122) You are a home health nurse caring for a patient who is managing diabetes. Part of your role includes helping this patient successfully manage their disease at home. You achieve this if you _________.

(A) Teach the patient to come in when there is any sign.

(B) Teach the patient home care strategies for the illness.

(C) Teach the patient danger signs and when to report to the hospital.

(D) B and C.

(123) During a community education session on substance abuse, you address misconceptions about the condition. You explain that one common misconception is that substance abuse _________.

(A) Is the overuse of addictive substances.

(B) Is the use of unprescribed substances.

(C) Can lead to physical dependence.

(D) Cannot happen without dependence.

(124) As a mental health nurse, you're assessing the support system available to a patient with a substance abuse problem. The tools you use to perform this assessment include ________.

(A) Interval follow-up evaluation, range of impaired functioning.

(B) CAGE-AID, drug abuse screening test.

(C) MAS test, CAGE-AID.

(D) All of the above.

(125) You are part of a disaster response team dealing with the aftermath of a massive earthquake where thousands of people are displaced and many lives lost. This is considered a(n) _______ crisis.

(A) Situational.

(B) Developmental.

(C) Adventitious.

(D) None of the above.

(126) As a nurse practitioner, you're preparing a presentation on Leininger's transcultural nursing theory. While discussing the components of this theory, you mention that it does not include ________.

(A) Cultural interference and restructuring.

(B) Cultural preservation and maintenance.

(C) Cultural care negotiation and accommodation.

(D) Cultural care repatterning and restructuring.

(127) You are a public health nurse who works with families dealing with different stressors. You explain that some factors that impact family functioning are biological needs, such as __________.

(A) Ill health.

(B) Disability.

(C) Unemployment.

(D) A and B.

(128) You are an inpatient psychiatric nurse who cares for a patient newly diagnosed with schizophrenia. When you educate the patient's family, you explain that schizophrenia belongs to the ________ class of mental illnesses.

(A) Psychotic disorder.

(B) Personality mental disorders cluster C.

(C) Personality mental disorders cluster A.

(D) Personality mental disorder cluster B.

(129) You are an ICU nurse who cares for a patient who exhibits a rapid heart rate, rapid breathing, and increased blood pressure. According to Hans Selye's theory, these physiological responses suggest the patient is in which stage of the stress response?

(A) Alarm.

(B) Resistance.

(C) Exhaustion.

(D) All of the above.

(130) As a mental health nurse, you're communicating with a patient who is already defensive and non-communicative. To promote therapeutic communication, you should avoid _______.

(A) Challenging.

(B) Clarification.

(C) Paraphrasing.

(D) Focusing.

(131) You're reviewing the medication list of a patient who has renal disease, is pregnant, and has a history of drug allergies. Knowing general contraindications to medications, all the following would be concerns except _______.

(A) Pregnancy.

(B) Renal disease.

(C) Allergies to the medicine.

(D) Reduced body weight.

(132) As a nurse, you're working with a team of physicians. When it comes to drug prescription for patients, your role does not include ________.

(A) Helping prescribe drugs to patients.

(B) Understanding the pharmacology of drugs and the pathology of the patient.

(C) Discussing concerns about a prescription with the ordering physician.

(D) Determining if the prescription is necessary based on the patient's pathology and the drug pharmacology.

(133) You're monitoring a patient who just received a new medication. You notice the patient begin to have trouble breathing. This symptom would classify as ________.

(A) Difficult breathing following drug administration.

(B) Visual impairment following drug administration.

(C) Lip swelling following drug administration.

(D) Phocomelia seen in infants resulting in short limbs after administration of thalidomide in pregnancy.

(134) As a preoperative nurse, you confirm a patient's blood type for possible transfusion during surgery. Knowing about blood types, which statement is incorrect?

(A) Blood type O is a universal recipient.

(B) Blood type AB is a universal recipient.

(C) Blood type O is a universal donor.

(D) AA is a common genotype.

(135) You are a nurse preparing to administer a blood product to a patient with a low platelet count. Of the following options, which one is not considered a blood product?

(A) Cryoprecipitate.

(B) Packed blood cells.

(C) Erythrocyte sediment.

(D) Platelets.

(136) As an ICU nurse, you're caring for a patient with a central venous line. In maintaining this line, it's important to know it should be flushed daily with ________.

(A) Heparin.

(B) Warfarin.

(C) Normal saline.

(D) Protamine.

(137) You're a pediatric nurse caring for a child who needs nutrition support due to severe malnutrition. The doctor decides to initiate nutrition support via a venous line. In this situation, you know that __________ should not be given through the venous line.

(A) Parenteral nutrition.

(B) Chemotherapy.

(C) Enteral nutrition.

(D) Blood.

(138) As a nurse, you're preparing to administer medications to your patients. In doing so, which of the following aspects is the most critical for ensuring patient safety?

(A) Understanding the conversion of different metric systems in mathematics.

(B) Understanding the relevant clinical metrics in drug administration.

(C) Estimating figures of dosages.

(D) Understanding brand dosage.

(139) You're calculating a patient's medication dosage. The doctor ordered 2 grams of a medication, but the medication on hand is in milligrams. What is the conversion factor between grams and milligrams?

(A) 1 gr = 100 mg.

(B) 1 gr = 10 mg.

(C) 1 gr = 1 mg.

(D) 1 gr = 1000 mg.

(140) You're a home health nurse caring for a patient who needs to learn several unique procedures. However, one of the following items doesn't need specific training. Identify it.

(A) Using an inhaler.

(B) Taking insulin.

(C) Administering tube feedings.

(D) Checking the medication label.

(141) Before administering a medication to a patient, you check the medication label. Which of the following should you confirm?

(A) Name of the medication.

(B) Dose of the medication.

(C) Expiry date of the medication.

(D) All of the above.

(142) You're a nurse discharging a 23-year-old student who has just recovered from an episode of severe acute asthma. What kind of training would be most beneficial for this patient?

(A) Inhaler technique.

(B) Taking insulin.

(C) Self-administering tube feeding.

(D) Giving intramuscular injections.

(143) You're caring for a patient on total parenteral nutrition. During your shift, you keep a close watch for complications, which include _______.

(A) Sleepiness.

(B) Vomiting.

(C) Diarrhea.

(D) Infection, sepsis, liver dysfunction, and metabolic imbalances.

(144) As an oncology nurse, you're caring for a patient with severe pain related to their condition. How can you help manage this patient's pain?

(A) Help the patient sleep.

(B) Distract the patient from the pain.

(C) Administer pain medication.

(D) Tell the patient to endure the pain.

(145) You're providing education to a patient about their pain management plan, which includes nonopioids. You explain that these medications are primarily used for _______.

(A) Mild pain.

(B) Moderate to severe pain.

(C) Chronic pain.

(D) Emotional pain.

(146) As a nurse, you're teaching a patient about the role of nonpharmacological pain management techniques, such as deep breathing and distraction. What would you tell the patient the main purpose of these techniques is?

(A) Provide immediate pain relief.

(B) Eliminate the need for pain medication.

(C) Distract patients from pain.

(D) Improve patient satisfaction.

(147) You're caring for a patient who is experiencing postoperative pain. When explaining the importance of pain management, you tell the patient that the primary goal is to ___________.

(A) Prevent patients from seeking medical attention.

(B) Avoid the need for pain medication.

(C) Promote patient comfort and well-being.

(D) Encourage patients to endure pain without intervention.

(148) A patient has been on opioid medications for chronic pain, but now the physician has decided to discontinue the medication. As the nurse, you explain to the patient that opioid medications should be discontinued ____________.

(A) Abruptly.

(B) When the patient requests it.

(C) Based on the healthcare provider's discretion.

(D) In a gradual and supervised manner.

(149) You're a nurse preparing to start intravenous therapy for a patient. When considering the best location for the IV, you would most likely choose the __________.

(A) Most distant veins on the nondominant hand.

(B) Hand veins.

(C) Upper limbs.

(D) Lower limbs.

(150) You're caring for a patient receiving intravenous therapy and are monitoring for potential complications. What are some signs that the patient may be experiencing fluid overload?

(A) Hematoma and phlebitis.

(B) Allergic reactions and anaphylaxis.

(C) Infections and emboli.

(D) Edema and respiratory distress.

Test 1: Answers and Explanations

(1) (C) Delivery of the fetus.

The second stage of labor is from full cervical dilatation (10 cm) to delivery of the fetus. Braxton-Hicks contractions occur during the first stage of labor, usually during the latent phase. Here, mild or minor contractions happen, but cervical dilatation is less than 4 cm.

(2) (D) B and C.

The nurse must assess the patient before arriving at the diagnosis and recognizing the patient's need. Once a need for referral is recognized, the RN should contact the appropriate external resource that can meet the needs of the patient. The external resources in the scenario presented are the psychologist, the psychotherapist, and the physician.

(3) (C) Young man, middle-aged man, teenager, elderly woman.

The nurse should prioritize patients based on the severity of their conditions. The young man who lost a lot of blood is in a life-threatening situation and should be attended to first. The teenager experiencing an adverse reaction from a blood transfusion should be second. Pain from osteoarthritis, while uncomfortable, is not immediately life-threatening, so the middle-aged man would be third. The elderly woman would be last because she is coming in for routine chemotherapy.

(4) (C) "I am sorry, Joe. I can't give you that information."

Let Joe know that you cannot give out such information. HIPAA protects the patient's personal information, such as name, date of birth, social security number, diagnosis, and treatment. This act ensures that those who have access to the information are involved in the management or care of the patient.

(5) (D) "I cannot give the medication because you did not document it. Verbal orders are recognized only during emergencies. I suggest you ask another physician to come document it."

Verbal orders should not be used except in case of emergency, and a nurse is one of those responsible for maintaining order in the healthcare setting. If an order is given and not documented and anything goes wrong, the nurse will be liable because it was not documented. So, the question should be, "Who gave the order?"

(6) (A) Internal locus.

Locus of control refers to the point where an individual's control or power over the future lies. In some people, the locus of control is internal. In others, it is external. When it is internal, individuals believe they have control over their own future and whatever troubles they might encounter. When it is external, individuals believe that the future and all it brings is beyond their abilities to impact.

(7) (D) All of the above.

While the question does not provide specific details about the child's behavior, it mentions that the child has started to challenge the mother's authority at home. Given this information, it is important to counsel the mother on helping her child avoid potential risks. The options provided include smoking, unsupervised swimming, and falls. These are common risks that children may face, and it is essential to educate parents on how to prevent these hazards and ensure the child's safety.

(8) (A) Apologize to the patient and allow him to view his records.

Patients have a right to speak privately to their healthcare providers and have their information treated confidentially. They have the right to look through their medical records and request an amendment of any inaccurate information. You should apologize to the patient and allow him to view his records. Later, in private, you can speak to the staff about the rights of the patient.

(9) (D) CT scan.

Infections can present with a persistent fever that might resist antipyretics and tepid sponging. A blood culture might be required to detect the presence of microorganisms. A complete blood count would also be useful. A CT scan would not be routinely ordered for a patient with persistent fever.

(10) (D) EUCR, hyperkalemia.

Hyperkalemia is an elevation of the potassium levels in the blood above the expected standard value. Features of hyperkalemia include muscle paralysis, generalized body weakness, nausea, and cardiac arrhythmias. Therefore, this patient should be screened for hyperkalemia.

(11) (D) Visual assessment.

Patients with a long history of diabetes are more prone to visual abnormalities, such as cataracts, macular degeneration, and glaucoma, among other ocular conditions. This elderly patient potentiates the risk of visual abnormalities. Hence, the most appropriate assessment is a visual assessment. However, other basic care assessments should be carried out for all admitted patients.

(12) (B) Fecal impaction.

Fecal impaction is the collection of compressed or hardened feces in the colon or rectum, commonly occurring in older people. Prompt recognition and differentiation from other causes of the inability to pass stool are important in patient management.

(13) (C) Mobility issues can affect other systems aside from the musculoskeletal system.

Mobility issues can affect the respiratory, gastrointestinal, and urinary systems. Mobility issues can be from genetic or acquired factors. Muscle contraction is usually graded on a scale of 0 to 5. Mobility issues are usually multifactorial, involving nerves, muscles, electrolytes, and psychology.

(14) (D) Nonpharmacological comfort interventions can be effective in the management of pain.

Nonpharmacological comfort interventions, such as patient education, companionship, and music, can effectively manage pain. Acute pain is usually described based on duration and not severity. Pharmacological treatment is not always effective in pain management, and severe cases may need interventional rather than pharmacological management. Pain can be a complication of treatment in oncology cases. However, symptoms and resolution of pain can usually be a sign of improvement following treatment.

(15) (C) Document for possible revision of medications and reduction of dosage.

Documentation for possible medication revision and dosage reduction is the next best course of action, as overdosing can cause excessive somnolence. Other answer options are inaccurate.

(16) (B) Use of a waterbed.

The use of a waterbed is most appropriate for this patient to prevent pressure sores due to the severe injuries limiting mobility. Other options will not prove as effective or may further worsen the patient's condition.

(17) (D) Suprapubic (bladder) massage.

Suprapubic (bladder) massage will not increase the rate of renal elimination of the toxic substance.

(18) (A) Increased intravenous fluid intake.

Increased intravenous fluid intake is not an appropriate part of the evaluation and care of this patient as it offers little care for the primary pathology unless other complications, such as dehydration, occur.

(19) (D) Encourage ambulation.

Encouraging ambulation is an inappropriate line of care for this patient. Other options, such as the administration of antipyretics, tepid sponging, adequate exposure and increasing fluid intake, all aim to reduce the body temperature.

(20) (A) Sedate the patient.

Sedating the patient is an inappropriate line of care as it will affect the assessment of consciousness and mask neurological signs needed for patient evaluation. All other lines of care are appropriate for this patient.

(21) (D) Regular fasting.

Regular fasting is not advisable for this patient, who has previously been diagnosed with an eating disorder. All other counsel will benefit the patient and is adjuvant care in managing cholecystitis.

(22) (B) Spoon-feed the patient while propped up in bed.

Spoon feeding the patient while the patient is propped up in bed poses a high risk of aspiration.

(23) (B) History of maternal illness in pregnancy.

The history of maternal illness in pregnancy is the most inappropriate question in the evaluation of this patient as the child is past the neonatal period, and poor weight gain is likely related to the current diet and acquired factors.

(24) (A) Zimmer's walking frame.

Zimmer's walking frame is the best mobility assistive device for this patient as weight is evenly distributed and weight bearing on the post-op limb is reduced.

(25) (B) Addiction.

Addiction is the constant need for a person to take a particular substance despite obvious physical, mental, and social or economic harm and a loss of control over the use of that substance. So even though Matt knows his smoking is affecting him, he still feels a need to keep smoking.

(26) (B) Evaluate the patient using CAGE-AID.

CAGE-AID is a standard test for evaluating patients with substance abuse disorder. Patients in this category might display hyperactivity or slow movements, tremors, poor hygiene, the presence of needle marks on upper and lower extremities, and poor health status.

(27) (D) All of the above.

Needs might be adequate nutrition and fluids due to anorexia and dehydration. Patients might also have psychological needs that can be diverse. Some of these can be corrected, while others might have to be managed with the help of psychologists and family members.

(28) (A) Denial.

The Kübler-Ross model describes grief in five stages: denial, anger, bargaining, depression, and acceptance. Denial is when the person refuses to accept the loss that has occurred.

(29) (D) B and C.

A nurse must attend to patients with a consciousness of their spiritual leanings and provide appropriate care for them without offending them.

(30) (C) Stop the transfusion, give normal saline, and inform the doctor.

In case of a transfusion reaction, the best response is to stop the transfusion and give IV normal saline. Antihistamines and corticosteroids with antipyretics can also be given, and urine output should be monitored. A doctor should be informed. It is important to send a blood sample from the contralateral limb of the patient for regrouping and crossmatching.

(31) (C) Hemolytic transfusion reaction.

People with blood type O are universal donors and can give blood to any type, but they are only compatible to receive blood from other type O donors. If a person with type O blood receives type B blood, their body would identify the B antigens as foreign and would mount an immune response. This could result in a hemolytic transfusion reaction, where the immune system destroys the transfused blood cells. This is a serious and potentially life-threatening response. Therefore, ensuring blood compatibility is crucial in transfusions.

(32) (B) Reassure the patient and inform the doctor.

Reassure the patient and ask the doctor to determine the next line of action. It is a known fact that some medications irritate veins. Hence, they should be administered slowly, and the patient should be reassured. However, if pain persists after administration, the IV line should be removed and another one inserted.

(33) (C) Intravenous route.

The intravenous route will be the most appropriate route for resuscitation of this patient as it can deliver fluids directly to the child's system without the risk of vomiting, which would likely occur in the oral route.

(34) (D) Legal documentation on how patients should be handled if they are unable to communicate.

Advance directives refer to legal documentation that clearly states the wishes of patients about their care if they become unable or incapacitated to communicate. Some advance directives include living wills, healthcare proxies/durable power of attorneys for healthcare, and the Uniform Anatomical Gift Act.

(35) (D) All of the above.

If an individual has prepared advance directives, the nurse should document this in the patient's records. Other relevant healthcare personnel should be informed, and the directives should be strictly adhered to as occasions arise. If these documents have not been prepared, the nurse can counsel the patient on the need to prepare them.

(36) (B) Tasks that require a lower level of professional judgment.

The nature of the task will determine if it can be delegated. Some tasks involve patient needs that follow set routines and require lower levels of professional judgment and competence. Such tasks can be easily delegated. But there are other tasks that involve meeting the needs of patients who are in dynamic or unstable conditions. Here, there can be rapid changes that require quick judgment calls and higher competence. Such tasks should not be delegated.

(37) (B) Right person, task, circumstance, direction, supervision.

The right person asks: *Is this the person right for the task?*
The right task asks: *Is this a task to be delegated?*
The right circumstance asks: *What is the state of the patient?*
The right direction/communication asks: *Is there a clear and detailed explanation of the task to be performed?*
The right supervision asks: *Who will be held accountable for the outcome of this task?*

(38) (D) Retrospective reimbursement.

In the retrospective reimbursement system, healthcare facilities receive payments for the care they render based on the cost, and insurance companies pay for all the services irrespective of the cost.

(39) (A) Individualization.

The plan that is developed for each patient must be individualized based on the patient's condition and need. This means that a nurse cannot make general healthcare plans for patients, even when they have similar diagnoses. No two bodies are the same, and individuals will always be unique in their physiology, their reactions, actions, and adaptations.

(40) (D) All of the above.

All patients have a right to choose the healthcare provider they want. They also have the right to choose the type of healthcare plans that they want and those that they do not want. This bill allows them to accept or reject interventions, no matter how essential healthcare personnel know they are.

(41) (D) Take on multiple roles for effectiveness.

Advocacy to other staff means updating other nursing staff members about patient advocacy and how this role should be seamlessly integrated into their practice. It should also include documenting or orally communicating the patient's needs to other staff members. It includes utilizing advocacy resources efficiently. Playing multiple roles is not part of efficacy, as all healthcare personnel have specialized training.

(42) (D) Circulation, airway, breathing.

The ABCs of resuscitation mean airway, breathing, and cardiovascular or circulatory system. This is useful in deciding where to start attending to a patient who has undergone a cardiac arrest. However, it is crucial to note that the recent update has changed the sequence to CAB, meaning chest compressions come first, followed by airway and then breathing.

(43) (C) An environment where errors are viewed as opportunities for learning and improvement

A blameless or blame-free environment is required for performance improvement. A blameless environment is one where mistakes are seen as opportunities for improvement. In this type of environment, the focus is not on the individual who made a mistake but on the different ways to improve the processes and workflow and make it fail-safe.

(44) (A) Core measures.

Core measures refer to standard measurements of quality. They are developed by the JCAHO (Joint Commission on the Accreditation of Health Care Organizations). They evaluate values like the population of patients on the ward, specific diseases (such as pneumonia or sepsis) and organizational measures.

(45) (D) All of the above.

All methods of performance improvement have the following in common: problem definition, relevant data collection, analysis of collected data, root cause analysis, generating possible solutions or alternatives, narrowing down to a solution or alternative with the greatest feasibility and highest chance of success and evaluation of the effectiveness of the implemented solution.

(46) (B) Registered Nurses (RNs).

RNs are licensed healthcare personnel who are trained to deliver nursing care in healthcare settings. They can manage both stable and unstable patients in structured or unstructured environments. They are also trained to coordinate other nursing team members, such as nursing assistants and LPNs.

(47) (D) Social workers.

Social workers ensure that the patient is appropriately moved in the continuum of care and that there is no deficit after the patient is discharged. They are also essential in cases of child abuse, neglect, or malpractice and can provide a much-needed link and support for victims.

(48) (C) Conceptualization.

At this point, those affected by the conflict begin to understand what is happening and why it happened. They begin to provide logical or illogical reasons that they believe have brought them to that position.

(49) (C) Avoidance, accommodating without addressing issues, competition.

Avoidance: Prolonged withdrawal and avoidance of the entire situation are unhealthy.
Competition: Competition is very unhealthy for the healthcare team when it stems from conflict.
Accommodating others without addressing issues: Although it is good to be accommodating and considerate, issues that are important to the individual should be resolved.

(50) (C) Race.

Race has nothing to do with establishing priorities in patient care. Any racial discrimination is a crime and can make healthcare personnel liable for litigation. Racial discrimination is a very serious offense, and it is not tolerated in healthcare practitioners. Priorities should be based on an understanding of the pathophysiology of the disease condition and presentation to know who needs more urgent care.

(51) (C) The patient's recovery progress.

The ultimate determinant of the effectiveness of care is the recovery of the patient.

(52) (B) The ethical standards conflict with the patient's interests.

Many times, ethical dilemmas come into play when an action might be in the patient's interest but is not in line with ethical standards. Nurses must not have any clash of beliefs with ethical standards. Whatever opinions they have should have been addressed long before care is delivered to the patient.

(53) (A) The evaluations help nurses better fulfill their duties.

For nurses to understand their responsibilities, performance evaluations outcomes should be conducted. The quality of the care nurses provide to their patients must be assessed and reported for further research or review.

(54) (D) 09/12/20 1020 hrs. IM Diclofenac 75 mg STAT given. Patient reports pain level as 2/10.

The right way to input information for patients is the date, time, drug and correct route of administration, dose frequency, and assessment of the patient.

(55) (D) B and C.

Blind patients can hear, so they can be communicated with through speech. Braille is a system of reading and writing that utilizes tactile representation of letters of the alphabet using raised dots. Blind people or those with poor vision use it. In the healthcare setting, it can be used effectively to communicate with blind patients by those trained in its use.

(56) (D) B and C.

Target screening can be conducted when some people show strong tendencies, signs, or symptoms of a particular condition or disease. This target screening is also conducted when a patient is at risk of a certain ailment or the caregiver needs to rule out a possible condition.

(57) (D) Help patients express themselves more.

The purpose of a health history is to gather information about the patient's health status. This involves the use of open-ended questions (Option A) to gather broad subjective information, and closed-ended questions (Option B) to gather specific factual details. Interview-style questions (Option C) are often used in health histories to engage in dialogue with the patient. Therefore, these all are parts of a health history. However, a health history does not inherently help patients express themselves more (Option D), as it is focused on collecting information related to their health, not on improving their communication or self-expression skills.

(58) (D) All of the above.

A patient who has been having regular unprotected sex can be counseled on abstinence, sticking to a partner, or using condoms to reduce the risk of contracting STIs. Nurses can also counsel patients on the need to use contraception to prevent unwanted or unplanned pregnancies.

(59) (A) Educate the parents on the importance of a balanced diet.

Parents are usually responsible for feeding their children. Therefore, counseling the parents is very important to ensure a balanced diet for all family members.

(60) (D) All of the above.

Assessments can also be structured and have formal questions. They can be set surveys or interviews. Assessments can also be made by observing the behavior of patients.

(61) (B) Sensorimotor stage.

This stage also coincides with Piaget's first phase of cognitive development in children, known as the sensorimotor stage. Children learn about their surroundings through their sensory and motor activities at this stage.

(62) (A) Caring for children and aging parents.

Individuals in this stage are middle-aged adults. Adults at this stage are concerned with a need to produce structures, people, and things that will outlive them. They have various worries, ranging from childcare to aging parents' care. They are also concerned about diagnoses of chronic health conditions and worry about their impact on the world.

(63) (B) It affects how the body metabolizes prescription medications.

Hepatic changes will result in reduced hepatic blood flow and metabolism, leading to reduced hepatic clearance and a subsequent increase in the concentrations of medications in the body.

(64) (B) An ultrasound scan done in the first trimester of pregnancy.

The most accurate method of determining the EDD is through an ultrasound scan done in the first trimester of pregnancy. The LMP is limited because the mother might not recall the exact date, and the cycle might not be exact. Ultrasound done after the first trimester is not as accurate. The ovulation date is also not reliable.

(65) (C) Warm water.

Alcohol should not be used to clean the umbilical cord as it can irritate the skin, delay healing, and delay the stump from falling off. Warm water several times a day is now recommended. Other parts of the baby should also be cleaned.

(66) (D) All of the above.

Common allergic reaction symptoms include but are not limited to swelling, numbness, itching, or tingling at the exposure point; breathing difficulties; rashes or bumps; hypotension; and tachycardia. Swelling, numbness, or tingling sensations around the lips, mouth, or tongue usually indicate extremely serious allergic reactions.

(67) (B) Document the patient's allergic reaction for future reference.

Every allergic reaction must be documented to inform future healthcare measures. The substance that the patient reacted to, the dose of the substance and what was done to arrest the situation should be clearly documented. The patient should also be duly informed about what caused the reaction.

(68) (B) A 30-year-old patient who has been sedated and is unrestrained.

The 30-year-old sedated and unrestrained patient is more prone to falls and injuries than other patients. While factors, such as age and mental state, can make patients more prone to falls and injuries, other factors such as level of consciousness, muscular strength, and impaired reaction time are also high-risk factors.

(69) (D) Either 4'9" or 80 pounds.

Car seat laws and requirements for infants and children can vary by state. However, most laws require that infants and toddlers be strapped in car seats until they are 4'9" or 80 pounds.

(70) (B) Have oxygen and suction equipment readily available.

Preventive measures for patients at risk of seizures include identifying and removing environmental triggers, lowering the patient's bed or having the mattress placed on the floor, and having oxygen and suction equipment at the patient's bedside at all times.

(71) (C) Using a single unique identifier along with the patient's room number for easy identification.

It is recommended to have at least two distinct identifiers aside from the room number of patients. Room numbers in themselves should not be used as unique identifiers. Rather, nurses should consider using patients' full names, complete dates of birth, and other unique identification codes.

(72) (B) Yes.

RNs should verify the appropriateness and accuracy of each treatment order, especially when any appear out of place or questionable. Nurses should contact the healthcare personnel who have prescribed such treatment or procedure for proper verification.

(73) (A) Code Gray is the appropriate code for communicating an infant abduction.

This is false. Code Blue is a code name for cardiac arrest. Other common codes include Code Red for fire, Code Orange for a chemical spill, Code Pink for an infant abduction, and Code Gray for a hurricane, cyclone, or severe weather storm.

(74) (A) Using the back muscles when lifting heavy objects.

Use your arm and leg muscles to lift, not your back. Also, provide a secure base for supporting yourself while lifting by keeping your feet apart. The muscles of the back should not be used to lift.

(75) (D) The patient's height, weight, and muscular strength.

Every assistive device assigned to a patient must be properly suited to meet individual needs, such as cognitive ability, muscular strength, developmental stage, height, weight, and environment. Other factors, such as the distance of the patient's home, cultural and religious affiliations, and income level, do not play a significant role in determining the patient's ability to use an assistive device.

(76) (D) The intern disposes of biohazardous material in any available trash can.

Disposal of biohazardous material in any trash can is inappropriate and dangerous. A general principle for handling biohazardous waste is to properly dispose of it following stipulated national, state, and local laws.

(77) (D) All of the above.

Some situations nurses should look out for when inspecting equipment include frayed electrical cords, overloaded power outlets, loose or missing equipment parts, and other questionable conditions that could threaten the patient care environment.

(78) (C) Participation in periodic training and mock drills.

A key way for RNs to prepare for security threats is to go for periodic training and review policies and procedures for ensuring security before any breach occurs.

(79) (A) Airborne, contact, droplet, and vector-borne.

The mode of transmission is the specific medium through which the infectious agent is transmitted from the reservoir to a new host. Modes of transmission of pathogens are contact (direct and indirect), airborne, droplet, and vector-borne. When pathogens leave through the portal of exit of a reservoir, they are borne through these mediums until they gain access to the portal of entry of a new host.

(80) (C) Getting bitten by a mosquito carrying the West Nile virus.

Vector-borne transmission occurs when an insect or other animal spreads a pathogen. In this case, the mosquito acts as a vector, carrying the West Nile virus from one host to another.

(81) (D) All of the above.

Handwashing should be done before and after contact with a patient; before and after removing gloves; after touching equipment, instruments, and other treatment materials with bare hands; and when hands have been soiled with bodily fluids, secretions, and chemicals.

(82) (A) Measures taken to prevent the transfer of disease-causing organisms from one person or object to another.

Aseptic techniques are measures taken in addition to standard and transmission-based precautions to prevent the transfer of disease-causing organisms from one person or object to another. Aseptic techniques include barriers, patient and equipment preparation, environmental controls, and contact guidelines.

(83) (B) Reports should go to the Centers for Disease Control and Prevention.

Reports about communicable diseases, epidemics, and other outbreaks should be submitted to the Centers for Disease Control and Prevention.

(84) (B) Ensure all staff members strictly adhere to infection control measures.

RNs should watch out for themselves and other staff members to ensure they adhere to good infection control and prevention measures.

(85) (A) The patient's level of consciousness.

Every restraint or safety device used must be appropriate for every situation and should not increase the risk of accidents or harmful situations. It's important to consider the patient's level of consciousness to ensure that the restraint or safety device doesn't cause further harm.

(86) (D) Body Mass Index (BMI).

A patient's vital signs include blood pressure, pulse rate, respiratory rate, and body temperature. These four signs signify the body's most basic functions. The Body Mass Index (BMI) is a measure of the body's weight-to-height ratio. It is used to divide people into normal, overweight, and obese.

(87) (A) Korotkoff sounds.

Korotkoff sounds are produced by the blood pressure cuff and heard with a stethoscope when checking for blood pressure. They are produced as the cuff compresses the brachial artery and causes turbulent blood flow in the artery. The sounds are divided into five phases.

(88) (D) A and B.

Before performing any test, it is necessary to confirm the doctor's order for the tests and that the right patient is getting the test. This can be done by checking the order that was documented by the doctor. The next step is to ask the patient to say their name and then crosscheck that it is the same patient that the order was written for.

(89) (A) Electrical impulses of the heart.

The ECG records the electrical activities of the heart. It shows the velocity of the heartbeat, its consistency or rhythmicity, and how strong the electrical impulses are as they move from chamber to chamber in the heart.

(90) (D) None of the above.

All the methods listed can be used to obtain blood samples. Arterial sampling collects blood from arteries, venipuncture obtains blood from superficial veins, and a finger prick obtains blood from the fingertips.

(91) (D) Needle prick.

Venipuncture is a routine procedure carried out in the hospital. However, it has its complications. The patient is at risk of infection from a contaminated cannula. There's also the risk of injury to the skin, excessive bleeding, and delayed wound healing. The nurse is at risk of needle pricks. Needle pricks predispose nurses to infections such as hepatitis and retroviral disease.

(92) (B) Apply pressure on the sample collection site.

To prevent hematoma formation at the sample collection site during a venipuncture, pressure should be applied with gauze for a few minutes until blood flow stops. A hematoma happens when blood leaks from the vein into the surrounding tissues. It is most identifiable by swelling.

(93) (D) A conscious patient who recently underwent knee replacement surgery.

Patients with nasogastric feeding tubes are at risk of aspiration of oropharyngeal or gastrointestinal secretions. Patients with an impaired gag or cough reflex find it challenging to expel contaminants in the airway, so the contaminants stray into the lungs and block the airway. Sedated patients are also at risk of aspiration.

(94) (A) Hypovolemic shock.

Hypovolemic shock occurs when there is a depletion of blood fluids, which leads to a reduction in tissue perfusion. The endothelial cells experience ischemia because they are deprived of oxygen, and endothelial cell apoptosis occurs. The most common cause of hypovolemic shock is hemorrhage.

(95) (D) All of the above.

Patients who are malnourished and don't eat a balanced diet have a chance of skin breakdown because the nutrients to strengthen the connective skin tissues are absent. They also have a weak immune system and are prone to infections.

(96) (D) All of the above.

The quantity of drainage is measured and documented. The nature and color, if it is bilious or coffee-ground colored, might indicate that there is internal bleeding.

(97) (C) A few inches above the selected site.

The tourniquet is placed about four to five inches above the selected site. The purpose of the tourniquet is to block blood flow for a short period so that the vein is engorged and more visible for the insertion of the cannula.

(98) (C) A and B.

The catheter is inserted into the urethral meatus and advanced through the urethra above the point when urine is seen in the urine catheter. However, the catheter can also be inserted through the skin, at the pubic region into the bladder, by suprapubic cystostomy. This usually happens when the urethra is not patent.

(99) (B) Olfactory nerve.

The olfactory nerve is the first cranial nerve, and it is involved in smell. The nasal cavity contains more than 100 million olfactory receptors. These receptors are stimulated by molecules from different substances, then stimulate other fibers, which eventually stimulate the olfactory nerve.

(100) (C) Polydipsia.

Hypoglycemia commonly presents with lethargy, sweating, clumsiness, loss of consciousness, coma, and even death. Hyperglycemia presents with polydipsia (increased thirst) because there is an increased level of glucose in the blood. This increase leads to a high osmotic concentration of the blood, leading to dehydration, and this sends a signal to the brain to stimulate thirst.

(101) (A) Regional and general.

Anesthesia can be regional/local or general/systemic. Regional anesthesia is usually preferable because of the side effects and risks of general anesthesia.

(102) (B) Epidural.

Epidural anesthesia is a form of regional anesthesia where an anesthetic is injected into the epidural space above the dura mater. It is used during abdominal or lower limb surgeries or procedures. It is also given to women in labor who do not want to experience labor pains.

(103) (A) External.

External insults can be foreign bodies or microorganisms introduced into the body system from the exterior. External insults can result in internal injury. So, the gunshot is an external injury that eventually results in internal injury.

(104) (B) Breakdown of red blood cells (RBCs).

Bilirubin is formed from the breakdown of red blood cells. RBCs are broken down into heme and globin. Globin is broken into amino acids, while heme is further broken down into iron and biliverdin. The iron is reused and recycled, while the biliverdin is converted to the unconjugated form of bilirubin, which is transported to the liver bound to albumin.

(105) (D) All of the above.

Just like any procedure, the patient must give informed consent. The procedure must be thoroughly explained to the patient. The environment must be sterile, and aseptic techniques must be employed.

(106) (B) To reduce the breathing workload of the patient.

Ventilators reduce the breathing workload of the patient. The patient is intubated with an endotracheal tube that is appropriate for the age and procedure. The tube delivers the oxygen, which is also connected to the mechanical ventilator.

(107) (C) Artificial aspiration of pulmonary secretions.

Suctioning is the mechanical aspiration of pulmonary secretions from the airways. It is usually done in unconscious or sedated patients. Its purpose is to prevent secretions from blocking the airways or being aspirated into the trachea and lungs, which can lead to death.

(108) (D) None of the above.

Povidone is a good antiseptic, notable for drying wounds fast. Methylated spirit is useful for dressing, and honey has been noted to prevent bacterial infection and promote rapid healing, especially for open wounds. These all help to lower the rate of surgical site infection.

(109) (A) Take the patient's vital signs.

A patient recovering from general anesthesia is at risk of dysphagia and laryngospasms. The nurse monitors the patient after surgery. The vital signs are first taken. The pulse rate and blood pressure are measured. The respiratory system is also examined.

(110) (D) Coughing and postural drainage.

Simple techniques for pulmonary hygiene include coughing, deep breathing, and postural drainage. Advanced techniques include percussion and vibrations.

(111) (B) Openings from the outside to the inside.

Ostomies are surgical operations that create openings from the outside to the inside. They can be done to divert the bowels, such as through a colostomy.

(112) (A) Peritonitis.

Peritonitis is the inflammation of the abdominal cavity. Technically, it is the serosal membrane of the abdominal cavity and the organ it contains that is inflamed. It usually presents with fever, abdominal pain, diarrhea, ascites, and there might be ileus and diarrhea. There is also usually a history of recent abdominal surgery or previous history of peritonitis and immunosuppressive agents or diseases.

(113) (A) Upper limb.

The AV graft is a connection between an artery and a vein that is used in dialysis. The upper limb is the routine position for the graft, even though the lower limb can also be used when necessary.

(114) (D) Mercury.

Mercury is toxic to the human body. It is not an electrolyte. Sodium is the most dominant extracellular ion, and it helps in muscle contraction. Calcium helps with bone strengthening and cardiac contractions. Magnesium also plays a role in preventing the continuous contraction of muscles.

(115) (A) Diuretics.

Hyponatremia is the reduction in the sodium level in the body below the usual standard. Thyroid gland diseases, renal failure, and diuretic medications can cause hyponatremia. Both loop and thiazide diuretics are known to cause hyponatremia by inhibiting the absorption of sodium and stimulating sodium excretion, respectively.

(116) (C) Shock.

Hypovolemia is a reduction in the fluid in the blood. Hypovolemic shock occurs when there is a depletion of blood fluids, which leads to a reduction in tissue perfusion. This deficit in fluid in the blood volume and reduction of tissue perfusion can lead to shock, reduced cardiac output, coma, and death.

(117) (C) Ringer's lactate.

Blood volume expanders are intravenous fluids that can help to increase or maintain blood volume. They are usually important in conditions like hypovolemic shock or in surgery when there is anticipation of blood or fluid loss. Normal saline can also be used.

(118) (B) Continuous monitoring and recording of an ECG.

Telemetry is continuously monitoring and recording the ECG strips. It is mostly done by a telemetry technician, but nurses can monitor telemetry too.

(119) (B) Pneumothorax.

The patient's symptoms of shortness of breath and the chest not rising fully on one side are indicative of a pneumothorax, where air leaks into the space between the lung and chest wall. This leak causes the lung to collapse on the affected side, which impairs the mechanical function of breathing, leading to the noted symptoms.

(120) (C) A and B.

Arterial lines can be placed in the femoral, brachial, and radial arteries. These lines are inserted via a surgical procedure to monitor the patient's blood pressure. Arterial lines can also be used to obtain frequent blood samples.

(121) (A) Spirometry.

Patients with impaired ventilation/oxygenation should be assessed with pulmonary function tests, such as pulse oximetry, spirometry, lung compliance, and forced vital capacity.

(122) (D) B and C.

It is expedient that patients know what to look out for when they are at home. They should be able to recognize symptoms of a condition, what to do, and when to report to the hospital promptly.

(123) (D) Cannot happen without dependence.

Substance abuse is defined as the overuse of a substance that is addictive or use that is not prescribed by qualified medical personnel. Substance abuse can lead to physical dependence, which happens when a person begins to experience adverse physical reactions to drug withdrawal. However, it is important to state that addiction can occur without physical dependence.

(124) (A) Interval follow-up evaluation, range of impaired functioning.

Two standard assessment tools are interval follow-up evaluation and range of impaired functioning.

(125) (C) Adventitious.

An adventitious crisis occurs during a major social disturbance. It includes natural disasters, war, or terrorism. Developmental/maturational crises are predicted occurrences that happen in life. They occur due to growth. Situational crises refer to events that are unpredictable. They are random life events that happen to people.

(126) (A) Cultural interference and restructuring.

Leininger's transcultural nursing theory includes three major nursing decisions and actions:

Cultural preservation and maintenance help the patient retain and/or preserve relevant care values so they can maintain their well-being, recover from illness, or face handicaps or death.

Cultural care accommodation/negotiation helps the patient adapt to or negotiate with others for a beneficial or satisfying health outcome.

Cultural care repatterning/restructuring assists the patient to reorder, change, or greatly modify their lifestyle for new, different, and beneficial healthcare patterns.

Cultural interference and restructuring is not a component of Leininger's transcultural nursing theory, which makes it the correct answer.

(127) (D) A and B.

Ill health and disability are biological needs. Unemployment is a socioeconomic need.

(128) (A) Psychotic disorder.

Psychotic disorders include schizophrenia, schizotypal personality disorder, and schizoaffective disorder.

(129) (A) Alarm.

The stage of alarm is where certain physiological responses show that there is an upset in the body's homeostasis. The resistance stage is marked by increased cardiac output and a maintained respiratory rate and blood pressure increase. Here, the body is trying to deal with the effect of the stress. The third stage is exhaustion; at this point, the body has used all its resources in trying to deal with the stress.

(130) (A) Challenging.

This means forcing patients to defend their choices and opinions. It is nontherapeutic and should be avoided. Clarification, paraphrasing, and focusing are all therapeutic.

(131) (D) Reduced body weight.

Pregnancy, renal disease, and allergy are all general contraindications to medications; however, reduced body weight is not a contraindication, as the dose can be recalculated for weight.

(132) (A) Helping prescribe drugs to patients.

It is illegal for a nurse to prescribe medications for patients as only the doctor is licensed to do so, except in states where nurses have such licenses. It is important to understand the pharmacology and the patient's pathology as this will help determine if there is anything wrong with the prescription so it can be discussed with the doctor.

(133) (A) Difficult breathing following drug administration.

Difficult breathing is life-threatening as this can lead to tissue hypoxia and death. Visual impairment is a very serious challenge but is not immediately life-threatening. Lip swelling is minor, and phocomelia, though an adverse reaction, is not immediately life-threatening.

(134) (A) Blood type O is a universal recipient.

Blood type A has A antigens, and blood type B has B antigens. AB has both A and B antigens, so it is a universal recipient as it cannot be transfused to any other blood type except AB. Blood type O has neither A nor B antigens, so an agglutination reaction will not occur since there is no antigen to react with. Hence blood type O is a universal donor.

(135) (C) Erythrocyte sediment.

Erythrocyte sediment is a measure of an active inflammatory process. Blood products are therapeutic substances derived from blood. The different blood products and their components are red blood cells, platelets, fresh frozen plasma, albumin, clotting factors, cryoprecipitate, and whole blood.

(136) (A) Heparin.

Central venous lines should be flushed daily and after every use with heparin.

(137) (C) Enteral nutrition.

Enteral nutrition is taken by direct tubing to the intestine or can be ingested orally but is contraindicated for venous administration.

(138) (B) Understanding the relevant clinical metrics in drug administration.

There are different metric concepts in mathematics, but some have more clinical significance. Estimation can be helpful but sometimes dangerous; for example, in the administration of chemotherapy, the slightest increase in dose can be lethal.

(139) (D) 1 gr = 1000 mg.

When converting from grams (gr) to milligrams (mg), the conversion factor is 1 gr = 1000 mg.

(140) (D) Checking the medication label.

Patients are taught to check medication labels, but it's not a unique procedure that requires special training.

(141) (D) All of the above.

The nurse is expected to verify the medication's name, dose, expiry date, and technique for administering it before administration.

(142) (A) Inhaler technique.

The patient will benefit from learning the appropriate inhaler technique for maintenance therapy.

(143) (D) Infection, sepsis, liver dysfunction, and metabolic imbalances.

Total parenteral nutrition (TPN) is a method of delivering nutrition directly into the bloodstream when oral or enteral nutrition is not possible or insufficient. While TPN can be beneficial in providing essential nutrients to patients, it is not without potential complications. Complications associated with TPN include the risk of infection, which can lead to sepsis, as well as liver dysfunction and metabolic imbalances.

(144) (C) Administer pain medication.

Nurses help manage pain primarily by administering pain medications to patients.

(145) (A) Mild pain.

Nonopioids are nonnarcotic analgesics that are used to manage mild pain. They are not typically used for moderate to severe or chronic pain, which may require stronger analgesics such as opioids. Nonopioids reduce pain and inflammation; examples of non-opioid drugs include NSAIDs.

(146) (C) Distract patients from pain.

Nonpharmacological pain management techniques, such as deep breathing and distraction, do not typically provide immediate pain relief in the same way that medications can. Instead, they work by helping the patient focus their attention away from the pain, thus reducing its perceived intensity.

(147) (C) Promote patient comfort and well-being.

Proper pain management is important to promote patient comfort and well-being.

(148) (D) In a gradual and supervised manner.

Opioid medications are usually tapered or discontinued gradually and supervised to prevent withdrawal symptoms and other complications.

(149) (A) Most distant veins on the nondominant hand.

The most distant veins on the nondominant hand are the best for the nurse to use so that the patient can fully use the dominant hand.

(150) (D) Edema and respiratory distress.

Fluid overload can lead to edema (accumulation of excess fluids in the third space) and respiratory distress. Respiratory distress can result from the accumulation of fluids in the pleural space.

Test 2 Questions

(1) Your patient, Mr. Adams, recently passed away. His family members are in a dilemma as they're unsure if they can decide to donate Mr. Adam's organs. What document will allow them to do so?

(A) Living will.

(B) Uniform Anatomical Gift Act.

(C) Health care proxy.

(D) None of the above.

(2) Mrs. Patel, a 65-year-old patient, is trying to arrange all her healthcare-related documents. She brings up a document and wants to know if it is a legal document. You inform her that ___________ is not a legal document.

(A) Value history.

(B) Self-determination act.

(C) Health care proxy.

(D) Uniform Anatomical Gift Act.

(3) You're in the ER, where two critical cases have just come in simultaneously. The first is a 60-year-old stroke patient, Mrs. Smith, who is unconscious, and the other is Mr. Jones, a 25-year-old diabetic patient who is also unconscious and appears to be dehydrated. You're considering which tasks you can delegate to your nurse assistant. What will you do to the nurse assistant?

(A) Ask her to turn the stroke patient.

(B) Ask her to resuscitate the 25-year-old.

(C) Delegate both tasks.

(D) None of the above.

(4) As a nurse, you're discussing the case management process with a group of nursing students. One of the students asks you what actions are involved in case management. Which of the following is not involved?

(A) Development of health care plans.

(B) Implementation of health care plans.

(C) Evaluation of health care plans.

(D) None of the above.

(5) Your patient, Mr. Lee, is recently diagnosed with a heart condition. You're developing a comprehensive care plan for Mr. Lee. What do you need to consider in developing this plan?

(A) Diagnosis.

(B) Actual problems.

(C) Potential problems.

(D) All of the above.

(6) Mr. Thompson, a patient under your care, expresses concern about the confidentiality of his personal medical information. What law lets you reassure him that his personal information is protected?

(A) Patient's bill of rights.

(B) HIPAA.

(C) Informed consent.

(D) All of the above.

(7) Mrs. Rodriguez, a new patient, is trying to understand her responsibilities while being under your care. Which of the following is not her responsibility?

(A) Treat health care workers with respect.

(B) Pay medical bills.

(C) Provide inaccurate information about health status.

(D) None of the above.

(8) You're working with a recently diagnosed cancer patient, Mr. Harrison. In explaining your role as a nurse advocate, which of the following is not considered as your advocacy?

(A) Sensitization.

(B) Explanation of diagnoses.

(C) Education.

(D) Rejection or acceptance of interventions on behalf of the patient.

(9) Your patient, Mrs. Williams, needs to be referred to a physical therapist. What would be your first step in referring Mrs. Williams?

(A) Obtain necessary orders.

(B) Delegate.

(C) Assess the client.

(D) All of the above.

(10) You're in the ER during a particularly busy shift. You are responsible for triaging incoming patients. As an RN, what are the crucial skills that you can use during this process?

(A) Organization.

(B) Time management.

(C) Diagnosis.

(D) All of the above.

(11) You're overseeing a group of new nursing graduates, and one of them asks you about the essential skills required to manage their workload effectively. Which of the following are essential?

(A) Effective communication.

(B) Systematic manner of work.

(C) Knowledge of declining less urgent tasks.

(D) All of the above.

(12) Mr. Brown, a patient on your ward, was recently transfused with two pints of whole blood. After the second pint, he had a severe transfusion reaction. The student nurse on your team wants to understand what kind of event this is. Which of the following events explains what happened?

(A) Adverse drug reaction.

(B) Sentinel event.

(C) Auspicious event.

(D) Tragic event.

(13) As a charge nurse, you're leading a team meeting to discuss measures focusing on the length of stay of 30 patients admitted for the same illness on your ward. What is this type of measure called?

(A) Core measures.

(B) Outcome measures.

(C) Quality measures.

(D) Quantity measures.

(14) During an interdisciplinary meeting, you notice a young nurse struggling to effectively collaborate with other healthcare professionals. To enhance her collaboration skills, what would you recommend her to focus on improving?

(A) High level of professionalism.

(B) Sound judgment.

(C) Good communication skills.

(D) All of the above.

(15) During a staff meeting, you are explaining the importance of interdisciplinary conferences to the new nursing staff. Why are interdisciplinary conferences important?

(A) They support the holistic management of patients.

(B) They allow nurses to contribute to client care.

(C) They offer learning opportunities from other health care disciplines.

(D) All of the above.

(16) In your team, there is noticeable tension between two nursing colleagues. You note that both parties feel their needs are being sidelined or ignored. What stage of conflict best describes the situation?

(A) Action.

(B) Conceptualization.

(C) Anger.

(D) Frustration.

(17) After a few weeks, the ongoing conflict between two nursing colleagues has escalated. They have started responding to their frustrations and the conclusions they have arrived at. What stage of the conflict best describes the scenario?

(A) Resolution.

(B) Individuals responding to the frustrations and conclusions they have arrived at.

(C) Third-party intervention.

(D) All of the above.

(18) An unconscious young man, known to have type I diabetes, is rushed into the ER. You note that he has a fruity smell as you examine him. At this critical moment, what is the most important investigation to initiate?

(A) Random blood glucose test.

(B) Urine test.

(C) Complete Blood Count (CBC).

(D) Fasting blood glucose test.

(19) While caring for Mrs. Johnson, a patient with a complex medical history, her condition changes frequently. How often should the care plan be revised?

(A) Daily.

(B) Weekly.

(C) As often as needed.

(D) Seldom.

(20) As a nurse, you have often found yourself in situations where you had to make difficult decisions that involved ethical dilemmas. What should you express during a discussion with a nursing student?

(A) Ethical dilemmas can be avoided in nursing care.

(B) Ethical dilemmas cannot be avoided in nursing care.

(C) Adhering to ethical standards will never go against the client's interests.

(D) None of the above.

(21) As a nursing professor, you're teaching your students about the importance of the code of ethics in the nursing profession. What should you highlight as the primary function of the code of ethics?

(A) It provides a framework for decision making.

(B) It provides responsibility reminders for nurses.

(C) It controls the nurses' behavior.

(D) Both A and B.

(22) During a conference discussing global development and the nursing profession, the topic of the code of ethics comes up. As the lead speaker, what must you advocate for the nurses to do as global development occurs?

(A) Abandon the code of ethics.

(B) Revise the code of ethics.

(C) Revisit the foundations of nursing.

(D) Make the code of ethics a matter of personal conviction.

(23) As a nurse, you're demonstrating the correct way to document patient care to a group of nursing students. What should you write in the following example: "On 11/12/20 at 08:30 hrs, ____."

(A) Acetaminophen 900 mg STAT given. Pain has subsided.

(B) Acetaminophen 900 mg total dose given. Pain is reported as 2/10.

(C) Acetaminophen given. The patient is feeling better.

(D) IV acetaminophen 900 mg STAT given. The patient reports pain as 5/10.

(24) While reviewing a patient's charts at the nurses' station, a relative of another patient asks to see the health records of their friend, who is also in the hospital. What should you say to the person?

(A) "I cannot allow that!"

(B) "I am sorry, I cannot allow you to see that."

(C) "Speak to your friend about it."

(D) All of the above.

(25) A patient who is about to be discharged from the hospital asks to take a look at her medical records. In response to her request, what should you say?

(A) "Here they are; take a look."

(B) "Here is my password; check on the system."

(C) "I am not permitted to do that."

(D) "I will get you a copy from the records office."

(26) While reviewing a patient's orders, you see that a medication has been ordered to be given QDS. A student nurse asks you what QDS means. What should you say to the student nurse?

(A) It means: give medication as often as needed.

(B) It means: give medication 4 times daily.

(C) It means: give medication 3 times daily.

(D) It means: give medication twice daily.

(27) Mrs. Davis, a patient on your ward, has just suffered a transient ischemic attack (TIA). When a nursing student asks you what actions would be considered negligence in Mrs. Davis's care, what should you explain?

(A) Admitting the patient is negligence.

(B) Administering alteplase is negligence.

(C) Not asking for a physiotherapist is negligence.

(D) Not evaluating the patient for stroke is negligence.

(28) As the charge nurse in a primary healthcare center, you're discussing target screening with your team. Which of the following would require target screening?

(A) A 45-year-old man presenting for his routine check-up.

(B) A 50-year-old man with acute rhinitis.

(C) A five-year-old boy whose weight for his age is below normal.

(D) Both B and C.

(29) During a role-play exercise in a nursing class, what should the instructor emphasize as that one critical trait that a nurse must display while taking a detailed history?

(A) Nonjudgmental behavior.

(B) Sentimental behavior.

(C) Attachment.

(D) Detachment.

(30) During a health education seminar at a local community center, you're discussing high-risk behaviors. Which of the following is not considered a high-risk behavior?

(A) Excessive sun exposure.

(B) Drug abuse.

(C) Lack of sleep.

(D) Exercise.

(31) During a nursing education seminar, you are discussing the concept of "readiness to learn." How many types does the concept have?

(A) 5.

(B) 2.

(C) 3.

(D) 4.

(32) A patient is scheduled for an appendectomy. Prior to surgery, what should the nurse instruct the patient to do?

(A) Avoid drinking or eating anything for eight hours before surgery.

(B) Take their regular medications the morning of surgery.

(C) Shave the surgical area the night before.

(D) Eat a light breakfast to maintain energy levels.

(33) You're supervising a maternity ward when a newborn is brought in. The child has an APGAR score of 6 at 1 minute. A new nurse asks you what this means for the child. Which of the following statements should you tell the nurse?

(A) Severely distressed, needs urgent intensive care.

(B) Moderately distressed, needs moderate resuscitation.

(C) In excellent condition.

(D) In good condition.

(34) While lecturing to a pediatric nursing class, you discuss Erikson's stages of psychosocial development. When explaining the second stage, known as "autonomy vs. shame and doubt," what should a nurse expect a child to do during this stage?

(A) Feed every two hours.

(B) Exhibit separation anxiety.

(C) Hop around.

(D) Master toilet training.

(35) You're leading a discussion in a high school health class about Erikson's stages of development. During the "identity vs. confusion" stage, what would be the unusual behavior for adolescents?

(A) Attraction toward the opposite sex.

(B) Decreased self-consciousness.

(C) Peer group acceptance.

(D) None of the above.

(36) As a geriatric nurse, you're educating a group of nursing students about what to expect when caring for elderly patients. Which of the following explains what one can anticipate among the elderly?

(A) Living retrospectively.

(B) A gradual decline in physical function.

(C) Seeking purpose.

(D) Both A and B.

(37) During a childbirth education class, you are reviewing the stages of labor with expectant parents. While discussing the active management of the third stage of labor, which of the following is not a part of it?

(A) 10 IU oxytocin.

(B) Controlled cord traction.

(C) Uterine massage.

(D) Placenta separation.

(38) You're a labor and delivery nurse preparing a room for a patient in labor. A nursing student asks you what equipment is used to monitor the fetal heart rate. What will you primarily use?

(A) A sphygmomanometer.

(B) A fetal heart Doppler.

(C) An ultrasound scan.

(D) All of the above.

(39) While monitoring a laboring patient, which is one major indicator of fetal distress during labor?

(A) An elevated fetal respiratory rate.

(B) Decreased fetal movement.

(C) Decreased uterine contractions.

(D) An elevated fetal heart rate.

(40) In a case study review with your team of nurses, you discuss a 35-year-old patient, gravida 4, para 0, 4 alive, who was presented with significant blood loss following a spontaneous vaginal delivery (SVD). The estimated blood loss exceeded 500 mL. What condition is indicated based on this data?

(A) Disseminated intravascular coagulation.

(B) Postpartum hemorrhage.

(C) Postpartum psychosis.

(D) All of the above.

(41) During your first shift at a new nursing facility, your charge nurse asks you to assess the client care environment. Which of the factors should be considered?

(A) Luxury and distance.

(B) Age and income level.

(C) Comfort and safety.

(D) All of the above.

(42) A nurse is providing postoperative care for a patient who underwent a total knee replacement. The patient's leg is swollen and warm to touch. What should the nurse suspect?

(A) A normal response to surgery.

(B) Infection.

(C) Deep vein thrombosis (DVT).

(D) Wound dehiscence.

(43) During a staff meeting at your hospital, the topic of promoting staff safety arises. How can staff nurses promote and achieve safety?

(A) Provide education and training.

(B) Create a safe and ideal work environment.

(C) Encourage staff communication.

(D) All of the above.

(44) You are supervising a group of student nurses during their clinical rotation. You're teaching them about care for immobile patients. How often should they turn clients who are unable to change their positions by themselves?

(A) Every 12 hours.

(B) Every two hours.

(C) Every hour.

(D) Every six hours.

(45) You are leading a training seminar on patient safety and discuss potential risk scenarios. You ask the group to identify which of the following clients could be at a higher risk of identification errors. Which is correct?

(A) An unconscious patient.

(B) A client in a public ward housing more than two patients.

(C) A patient whose name and last name are the same.

(D) A patient who cannot communicate in English.

(46) As the head nurse in the emergency department, you are preparing your team for potential disaster situations. When should nurses be prepared to handle emergencies?

(A) Only when they are internal disasters.

(B) Especially when they are disease outbreaks.

(C) Irrespective of where they occur and who is affected.

(D) When their clients are at high risk of being impacted, whether at home or in the client care environment.

(47) In a case review session with your team of nurses, you discuss patient discharge policies. Which client category should the nurses first recommend for discharge after treatment?

(A) Unstable clients.

(B) Ambulatory clients.

(C) Conscious clients.

(D) Clients in pain.

(48) During a disaster drill, you remind your staff about the importance of maintaining effective but discreet communication during disasters and emergencies. Why is this necessary?

(A) It prevents sabotage and further risks to those affected.

(B) It prevents the clients from understanding the gravity of their health situation and becoming worried.

(C) It prevents families and friends from becoming aware of the critical health situation of their loved ones.

(D) All of the above.

(49) While educating your nursing team on safety protocols, you discuss various types of hazardous materials. What is a hazardous material?

(A) Nonbiological material that poses no harm to living beings.

(B) Biological material that poses harm to living beings.

(C) Nonbiological material that poses some form of harm to living beings.

(D) Biological material that poses no harm to living beings.

(50) You are conducting a workshop on radiation safety for your oncology nursing team. You ask about the three major ways to ensure safety during radiation therapy. Which of the following is correct?

(A) Time, distance, and shielding.

(B) Handwashing, distance, and shielding.

(C) Disinfecting, distance, and shielding.

(D) Disposal, distance, and time.

(51) You are presenting a workshop on home health nursing. During the session, you ask to identify the role of nurses in ensuring client home safety. Which of these choices are correct?

(A) They assess the need for home modifications.

(B) They provide clients with home modification solutions.

(C) They educate clients on safety issues.

(D) All of the above.

(52) As part of a training module on home health nursing, you've created a case study where a nurse is assessing a patient's home for safety. What is a crucial factor that the nurse should consider when assessing client home safety?

(A) Distance to the health care facility.

(B) Slip-proof floors.

(C) Number of stories.

(D) Weight of the patient.

(53) During a staff meeting at the hospital, you are discussing the handling and labeling of hazardous materials. How should hazardous materials be labeled?

(A) With labeling that provides specific information for identifying the nature of each hazardous material.

(B) No label.

(C) With a label that indicates danger but does not provide any specific information about the nature of the risk involved.

(D) With a red label for easy recognition of danger.

(54) As the charge nurse, you are discussing hospital policies on incident reporting with a new group of nurses. Who should receive reports for incidents and other irregular occurrences?

(A) Clients and their family members.

(B) The supervising or charge nurse and the risk management department.

(C) Other health care personnel and patients.

(D) All of the above.

(55) During a training session on patient safety, you present a scenario in which a nurse is inspecting a piece of equipment. You ask the trainees why it is important to inspect equipment for safety hazards. Which of the following is correct?

(A) It ensures that the equipment is functioning properly.

(B) It prevents hazards, client complications, and injuries.

(C) It reduces the cost of equipment maintenance.

(D) It identifies potential legal liabilities.

(56) In a simulated scenario during a training session, you present a situation where a nurse encounters a piece of malfunctioning equipment. What should the nurse do?

(A) Dispose of the equipment immediately.

(B) Move the equipment to another client care area.

(C) Report and remove the equipment from the client care area.

(D) Attempt to fix the equipment so it can continue to be used.

(57) During a professional development seminar, you're discussing infection control measures with your colleagues. You ask them to identify the standard precautions. Which of these statements is correct?

(A) These are preventive and infection control measures used to combat and inhibit the spread of specific infections.

(B) These are measures taken to prevent the transfer of disease-causing organisms from one person or object to another.

(C) These are control measures used to prevent the spread of infection among clients, whether or not they've been diagnosed with any infection.

(D) These are specialized equipment used to protect specific body areas from injury and exposure to infectious agents.

(58) At a healthcare providers' conference, you participate in a panel discussion on infection control. You asked the panel and the audience about the most effective procedure for preventing the spread of infection in health care environments. Which of the following should be the answer?

(A) Wearing protective gloves.

(B) Proper hand hygiene.

(C) Disinfecting with bleach and other chemicals.

(D) Using sterile equipment.

(59) You are training a group of new nurses on surgical procedures. Which of the following is an incorrect statement about maintaining a sterile field?

(A) Wetness on the sterile field is acceptable.

(B) Staff working directly on the sterile field do not need to wear sterile masks.

(C) Nurses can turn their back to the sterile field.

(D) All of the above.

(60) During a performance evaluation meeting, you are discussing the importance of aseptic techniques with your nursing team. What is the purpose of evaluating and monitoring the aseptic technique staff members use?

(A) It ensures that the technique is in line with generally accepted procedures.

(B) It can fire staff members who do not use the technique correctly.

(C) It gives staff members a sense of autonomy.

(D) All of the above.

(61) You're a pediatric nurse preparing to conduct a health check for a one-year-old baby. What is the expected respiratory rate for a one-year-old compared to an adult?

(A) Higher respiratory rate.

(B) Lower respiratory rate.

(C) Similar respiratory rate.

(D) None of the above.

(62) As an emergency room nurse, you are taking care of a 26-year-old male known patient with a history of substance abuse. In your education session about the dangers of opioid addiction, you discuss the major risks. Which of the following is one of the major risks?

(A) Increased blood pressure.

(B) Increased body temperature.

(C) Depressed respiration.

(D) All of the above.

(63) You're training a group of newly recruited nurses about diagnostic tests. Which of these statements about diagnostic tests is incorrect?

(A) Materials should be by the patient's bedside before any diagnostic test.

(B) Consent is not really needed for noninvasive procedures.

(C) The procedures must be done aseptically.

(D) None of the above.

(64) As part of a training program, you are demonstrating how to perform a blood glucose test. After pricking the patient's finger, you apply pressure over the site of the needle prick. Why is this done?

(A) Homeostasis.

(B) Hemostasis.

(C) Static equilibrium.

(D) Aids wound healing.

(65) During a training session on phlebotomy, you asked your trainees to fill in the blank: "Venipuncture is the collection of blood from a __________." Which of the following should fill the blank?

(A) Superficial vein.

(B) Deep vein.

(C) Superficial artery.

(D) Deep artery.

(66) As a senior nurse, you're guiding a novice nurse on how to collect a patient's samples. Before taking any samples, what should the nurse do?

(A) Gather materials.

(B) Explain the procedure.

(C) Obtain consent.

(D) All of the above.

(67) You're giving a lecture on urine analysis to a group of nursing students. Which of the following is not assayed for in urine?

(A) RBCs.

(B) WBCs.

(C) Glucose.

(D) None of the above.

(68) As part of a health awareness campaign, you're preparing a seminar on the risks of smoking. You ask the participants about the kinds of cancers that are closely associated with smoking. Which of the following is correct?

(A) Esophageal.

(B) Skin.

(C) Brain.

(D) All of the above.

(69) As an oncology nurse, you're counseling a woman who is undergoing chemotherapy for breast cancer after a mastectomy. You discuss potential alterations due to the treatment. Which of the following is not a potential side effect that the patient should be prepared for?

(A) Back pain.

(B) Mouth sores.

(C) Nausea and vomiting.

(D) Weight changes.

(70) During a seminar for healthcare providers about invasive procedures, you ask the audience to identify the two main concerns associated with invasive procedures. Which of the following is correct?

(A) Cost, recovery.

(B) Infections, cost.

(C) Infections, bleeding.

(D) None of the above.

(71) You are an experienced nurse preparing to demonstrate to your team of newly hired nurses the procedure of inserting an NG tube into a patient. What is the first step to be taken before inserting an NG tube?

(A) Obtain informed consent.

(B) Do a quick X-ray.

(C) Inspect the nares.

(D) Hyperextend the neck.

(72) In a lecture you're giving to nursing students, you ask about the two types of intravenous access. Which of the following are correct?

(A) Central and parenteral.

(B) Parenteral and interosseous.

(C) Central and peripheral.

(D) All of the above.

(73) You're a nurse supervisor overseeing a procedure involving urinary catheter insertion. You notice a rookie nurse preparing to insert the catheter incorrectly. Which of the following statements is incorrect about urinary catheters?

(A) They can be used to void urine.

(B) They come in different sizes.

(C) Insertion is a sterile procedure.

(D) The patient should be in the prone position for catheter insertion.

(74) You are a neurology nurse, preparing to conduct a neurological system assessment on a new patient. Which of the following is not one of the assessments for the neurological system?

(A) Level of consciousness.

(B) Mental state examination.

(C) Muscle tone.

(D) Muscle length.

(75) In an exam scenario, a nurse educator poses a question to nursing students studying neurology: “Bell’s palsy affects the facial nerve. What symptoms would you expect to see in such a patient?”

What should be the answer?

(A) Inability to move hands and feet.

(B) Inability to make facial expressions.

(C) Inability to speak.

(D) All of the above.

(76) You’re a diabetes educator, giving a lecture about hyperglycemia. Which of the following is not a symptom of hyperglycemia?

(A) Polydipsia.

(B) Blurred vision.

(C) Fatigue.

(D) None of the above.

(77) You are in an anesthesia seminar. The speaker asks the audience to identify some of the common side effects of general anesthesia. Which of the following is correct?

(A) Persistent headaches.

(B) Nausea and vomiting.

(C) Drowsiness.

(D) All of the above.

(78) As a nurse educator teaching about anesthesia, you ask the students as to what level can spinal anesthesia be administered. Which of the following is correct?

(A) L3/L4 vertebrae.

(B) L2/L3 vertebrae.

(C) L1/L2 vertebrae.

(D) Below S1 vertebra.

(79) You are leading a workshop on hypothermia management. You gave a scenario where a patient is presented with initial signs of hypothermia. Which mechanism is not a part of how the body initially deals with hypothermia?

(A) Vasodilation.

(B) Vasoconstriction.

(C) Shivering.

(D) Increased heat rate.

(80) You are the charge nurse at a neonatal unit where a newborn is being treated for jaundice using the blue light method. You train the new staff on the precautions to take. What are some precautions when using the blue light method to manage jaundice?

(A) Cover the baby's body with oil.

(B) Cover the baby's eyes.

(C) Ensure the baby is fully clothed.

(D) Ensure the light is far from the baby's skin.

(81) Imagine you are supervising a team of nurses assisting in a complex invasive procedure. Which of the following is not a part of their duties as a nurse assistant?

(A) Anticipate the next steps and make materials available at the request.

(B) Ensure all forms and documents are signed.

(C) Request an opportunity to perform an invasive procedure.

(D) Ensure that informed consent is obtained.

(82) You're conducting a seminar on ventilator use for newly graduated nurses. Which of the following is a known complication associated with the use of ventilators?

(A) Alveolar hypodistension.

(B) Oxygen toxicity.

(C) Life support.

(D) Reduced breathing workload.

(83) As a nurse on a respiratory care unit, you're teaching a new recruit about the suctioning procedure. Why do nurses perform preoxygenation during suctioning?

(A) To maintain the airways.

(B) To collapse the airways.

(C) To prevent alveolar overdistension.

(D) To help secretions come out more easily.

(84) You're discussing wound care with a group of nursing students. When examining a wound, what are the things that nursing students should look at?

(A) Size of the wound.

(B) Discharge.

(C) Color of the wound.

(D) All of the above.

(85) You're counseling a patient who is due for surgery next week. Which of the specific complications should a patient try to avoid after surgery?

(A) Post-dural puncture headache (PDPH).

(B) Anemia.

(C) Hypoglycemia.

(D) Medication.

(86) During a staff training session, you ask your team on how they should position the patient if they want to drain the posterior bronchus of the lungs. Which of these is the right way to do it?

(A) Place the patient supine with the head of the bed elevated at 45 degrees.

(B) Place the patient prone with the head of the bed elevated at 45 degrees.

(C) Have the patient sit at 45 degrees.

(D) Have the patient lie down flat.

(87) As the nurse manager of a surgical unit, you are orienting new nurses on their roles in managing patients with ostomies. What roles will they play in the management of these patients?

(A) Routine care.

(B) Surgical site examination.

(C) Tube inspection for patency.

(D) All of the above.

(88) As a dialysis nurse educator, you are teaching nursing students about the vascular access used in hemodialysis. What is an arteriovenous (AV) fistula?

(A) It is a connection between two arteries.

(B) It is a connection between two veins.

(C) It is a connection between an artery and a vein.

(D) It is a connection between capillaries and arterioles.

(89) As part of a quiz on hemodialysis, you ask the students when an AV fistula should be created for a patient requiring dialysis. Which of the following is correct?

(A) At dialysis.

(B) After a week of dialysis.

(C) Three months before dialysis.

(D) Immediately after dialysis.

(90) During an anatomy and physiology lesson, you present a question on which electrolyte is most abundant within the human cells. Which of the following is the correct answer?

(A) Potassium (K).

(B) Sodium (Na).

(C) Calcium (Ca).

(D) Phosphorus (P).

(91) You are caring for a patient who has been vomiting and experiencing diarrhea for the past five days. Based on your knowledge of electrolyte balance, what is the patient at risk for?

(A) Hyperkalemia.

(B) Hypercalcemia.

(C) Hypomagnesemia.

(D) Hypokalemia.

(92) As a part of a lecture for nursing students on electrolyte disorders, you ask about the following conditions one might expect to see hypernatremia. Which of the following is correct?

(A) Cushing's disease.

(B) Diabetes mellitus.

(C) Diabetes insipidus.

(D) All of the above.

(93) In a trauma unit, you are teaching a new nurse about fluid balance. Which of the following is a common cause of hypovolemia in adults?

(A) Bleeding from trauma.

(B) Acute diarrhea.

(C) Fluid overload.

(D) Gluttony.

(94) During a training session for ICU nurses, you're discussing the concept of hemodynamics. Which of the following is not involved in the study of hemodynamics?

(A) Study of blood flow through the vessels.

(B) Study of factors responsible for the free flow of blood in vessels.

(C) Study of turbulent flow of blood in vessels.

(D) None of the above.

(95) In a simulation exercise, you're role-playing with a nursing student who's caring for a patient with an arterial line. What are your roles as a nurse in this situation?

(A) Monitor the hemodynamic status.

(B) Check for complications.

(C) Perform other routine care.

(D) All of the above.

(96) As a cardiac nurse educator, you're conducting a quiz with your nursing team. You ask which of the following tasks is not included in caring for a patient with a pacemaker. Which of these answers is correct?

(A) Assess the insertion site for bleeding.

(B) Place the patient on bed rest.

(C) Give support.

(D) Give anticoagulant medications.

(97) You are conducting a training session for telemetry nurses. Which of the following statements is false about monitoring an ECG?

(A) A telemetry technician can monitor the ECG.

(B) The nurse can monitor the ECG.

(C) Only the telemetry technician should monitor the ECG.

(D) All of the above.

(98) During a presentation on respiratory disorders, you ask the students which of the following is not a pulmonary function test. What should be the answer?

(A) Lung compliance.

(B) Spirometry.

(C) Forced vital capacity.

(D) Chest X-ray.

(99) In a case study discussion about patient care management, which of the following is false about a treatment plan?

(A) It includes education of the patient.

(B) It includes home care strategies.

(C) It does not include the financial implications of the treatment.

(D) It includes the financial cost of the treatment.

(100) You are caring for a patient admitted with heart failure secondary to hypertensive heart disease. The patient has been complaining of excessive and frequent urination and is currently on digoxin, furosemide, and lisinopril. As the nurse on duty, what should be your best next course of action?

(A) Stop medications immediately.

(B) Counsel the patient and allay his fears.

(C) Raise an alarm and inform the doctor on call.

(D) Pass a urinary catheter.

(101) During morning rounds, you visit Mrs. Johnson, a 60-year-old woman who had surgery to repair a large bowel perforation, with temporary exteriorization of the bowel loop to allow healing of the anastomosis. You need to explain to the new nursing students about the procedure done. Which option correctly explains it?

(A) Colostomy.

(B) Colectomy.

(C) Colotomy.

(D) Colonoscopy.

(102) Later in the day, you visit Mr. Davis, a 70-year-old man who was admitted following a cerebrovascular accident. While discussing his case with nursing students, what mobility issue should they not anticipate?

(A) Speech difficulty.

(B) Atelectasis.

(C) Bed sores.

(D) Muscle atrophy.

(103) In the afternoon, you encounter a 24-year-old high school student who is involved in a car accident and is currently being evaluated for pain management. You engage the nursing students in arranging the following options based on the WHO pain ladder management:

I. "Weak" opioid or multifactorial +/- non-opioid +/-adjuvant therapy

II. Interventional treatments +/- non-opioid +/- adjuvant therapy

III. Non-opioid +/- adjuvant therapy

IV. "Strong" opioid +/- non-opioid +/- adjuvant therapy

Which of these steps should be done in order?

(A) II, III, I, IV.

(B) III, I, IV, II.

(C) I, II, III, IV.

(D) IV, III, I, II.

(104) Later, you visit Mrs. Miller, an 80-year-old woman being managed for cerebrovascular accident. Which of the following sites is not a common area for pressure sores associated with immobility?

(A) Heels.

(B) Elbows.

(C) Knee.

(D) Scapula.

(105) During night shift, you review the sleep diary of a patient being managed for chronic insomnia who is on sleeping medications. To evaluate the quality of his sleep, which of the following statements best indicates his improvement?

(A) Patient slept for a longer period overnight.

(B) Patient feels refreshed after waking up.

(C) Patient tosses and turns a lot while sleeping.

(D) Patient has several dreams while sleeping.

(106) The following day, you are caring for a patient who had an exploratory laparotomy for a bowel perforation and has delayed healing of the abdominal incision site. Which of the following nutritional deficiencies is not closely related to this situation?

(A) Vitamin C deficiency.

(B) Vitamin E deficiency.

(C) Zinc deficiency.

(D) Low serum protein.

(107) As you continue your rounds, you visit a patient chronically immobilized in bed due to a debilitating illness. During the patient's care plan discussion, you ask to identify an intrinsic risk factor related to pressure sores in this patient. Which of the following correctly describes it?

(A) Adequate oxygenation.

(B) Elevated blood pressure.

(C) Poor turning in bed.

(D) Poor tissue perfusion.

(108) In the ICU, you're caring for an elderly patient who has been placed on total parenteral nutrition following a bowel resection for colon cancer. What is the best route of venous access for this mode of nutrition?

(A) A central venous catheter.

(B) A peripheral sited intravenous line with an 18-gauge cannula.

(C) An intraosseous line.

(D) A peripheral sited intravenous line with a 22-gauge cannula.

(109) In the pediatric unit, you're assessing a nine-year-old boy admitted for muscular dystrophy. During your assessment, the boy can lift his limbs from side to side but not against gravity. How would you score his muscle power on a scale of 0 to 3?

(A) 0.

(B) 1.

(C) 2.

(D) 3.

(110) During the admission of a new patient, you're supervising a nurse who's conducting the health assessment. You ask her, "What is not a component of a detailed health assessment?"

What should be her response?

(A) Limited physical examination.

(B) Detailed management plan.

(C) Thorough medical history.

(D) Appropriate investigation.

(111) You are on the night shift at the hospital when a patient under your care passes away. As you speak with the grieving family, you used the Kübler-Ross model to guide them through the grieving process. Which of the following is not a stage in the Kübler-Ross model of grief?

(A) Denial.

(B) Acceptance.

(C) Depression.

(D) Bereavement.

(112) As part of a multidisciplinary team caring for a child with cerebral palsy, you attend weekly meetings to discuss the child's progress and treatment plan. In one of these meetings, you discuss the necessity of various roles within the team. Which of these roles may not be necessary?

(A) A pediatric neurologist.

(B) A neurosurgeon.

(C) An occupational therapist.

(D) A nutritionist.

(113) During a physical assessment of a 15-year-old boy who uses a single-elbow crutch due to an iatrogenic injury to the sciatic nerve, you observe his walking pattern. Based on his medical history, what type of gait is he most likely to demonstrate?

(A) High steppage gait.

(B) Waddling gait.

(C) Antalgic gait.

(D) Festinant gait.

(114) Ray, a patient in your care, has been given a prescription for post-operative pain. Twice now, he has returned before the prescription is due to run out, claiming that he lost the medication. What would you suspect is going on based on this behavior?

(A) Withdrawal symptoms.

(B) Drug-seeking behavior.

(C) Physical dependence.

(D) All of the above.

(115) You're conducting a lecture for a group of nursing students on patients' reactions to a new diagnosis. You ask them how patients generally react when diagnosed. Which is the most likely response?

(A) Some are defensive.

(B) Some are aggressive.

(C) Some mask their low self-esteem.

(D) All of the above.

(116) You're creating a treatment plan for a 20-year-old male patient in your care who is dealing with sexual addiction. Which of the following options do you propose as potential interventions?

(A) Impulse control counseling.

(B) Cognitive-behavioral therapy.

(C) Medications.

(D) All of the above.

(117) A patient is recovering from general anesthesia after a hernia repair. What is the nurse's first priority?

(A) Check the surgical site for bleeding.

(B) Assess the patient's level of pain.

(C) Monitor vital signs.

(D) Assess for airway patency.

(118) A 50-year-old man with a history of suicidal attempts is brought to the ER exhibiting depressive symptoms. He appears detached and calm. In his current state, what should a nurse be most cautious about?

(A) Tendency to abuse medications.

(B) Tendency to inflict self-harm or harm others.

(C) Tendency to escape from the hospital.

(D) All of the above.

(119) A patient arrives in the ER accompanied by her family. Despite your attempts to communicate with her, she refuses to speak and continually redirects you to a male figure she identifies as "the head." How do you handle this situation?

(A) Quickly apologize and speak to the head.

(B) Insist on speaking to the patient.

(C) Educate the family on women's empowerment and rights.

(D) Refer the patient.

(120) You're conducting an in-service training on end-of-life care. You want to highlight the essentials of this type of care. Which of the following is not typically part of end-of-life care?

(A) Ensure that the patient is comfortable.

(B) Pain medications.

(C) Massage therapy.

(D) Assessment of discipline techniques.

(121) In your lecture to nursing students about family dynamics, you presented a case of a family where each member is allowed to make decisions without much input or control from the leaders. You ask the students to identify the type of family structure in this example. What is the correct answer?

(A) Authoritarian.

(B) Laissez-faire.

(C) Democratic.

(D) None of the above.

(122) During a bereavement support group meeting you are facilitating, you discuss various models of grief. You ask the group to tell you the components of Worden's tasks of mourning. Which of the following is correct?

(A) Accepting the loss, coping, altering the environment, resuming a healthy life.

(B) Shock and disbelief, awareness, restitution, resolution, idealization.

(C) Shock, awareness of loss, conservation withdrawal, healing.

(D) Denial, anger, depression, acceptance.

(123) As part of an in-service training on mental health, you present a case study of a man who has been exhibiting unusually grandiose behavior and making unrealistic claims about his political status. He appears highly excitable and insists he is perfectly fine. What is the most likely diagnosis for this patient?

(A) Bipolar disorder.

(B) Personality disorder.

(C) Depressive disorder.

(D) Anxiety disorder.

(124) In a community health discussion focused on occupational health, you discuss the risks associated with different types of jobs. When talking about remote workers, you ask what occupational health concern is most relevant to them. Which of the following is the most likely response?

(A) Commuting for long hours.

(B) Sitting for long hours.

(C) Standing for long hours.

(D) All of the above.

(125) You're tutoring a group of nursing students studying Hans Selye's theory of stress response. You asked at what stage of this theory does a patient experience increased cardiac output. Which is correct?

(A) Alarm.

(B) Resistance.

(C) Exhaustion.

(D) Both A and B.

(126) During an intake interview, your client enthusiastically shares stories about his wife but neglects to provide needed information about his previous medications. Which of the statements can help you steer the conversation back to the necessary topic?

(A) "Please, can we discuss the medications now?"

(B) "Thank you so much for telling me about your wife. I am sure she is an amazing person. But can we also discuss your medications, so we can get you back home to be with her soon?"

(C) "I would prefer we discuss the medication now. Your wife is not the reason you are here."

(D) "I understand you miss your wife. But we need to get this over with the medications."

(127) During an allergy awareness presentation at a local community center, you want to dispel some common misconceptions about allergies. Which of the following statements about allergies is not true?

(A) Every human has an allergy.

(B) Signs and symptoms of allergic reactions vary per person.

(C) Allergic reactions can quickly become life-threatening.

(D) Not all allergens are life-threatening.

(128) In a clinical skills lab, you demonstrate the administration of IV medications to nursing students. You present a scenario where a patient is prescribed both IV calcium gluconate and IV sodium bicarbonate. What is the best method to administer these medications?

(A) Give both in quick succession.

(B) Give both slowly but immediately, one after the other.

(C) Give both within one hour.

(D) Give both one hour apart and flush the line in between both doses.

(129) During a blood transfusion education session for new nurses, you quiz them on what can be mixed with blood during a transfusion. Which of the following can be safely mixed with blood during a transfusion?

(A) Normal saline.

(B) Ringer's lactate.

(C) Acetaminophen.

(D) None of the above.

(130) As part of your pre-transfusion check, you discuss the necessary assessments to be made before starting a blood transfusion. Which of the following is not necessary?

(A) The religious or cultural beliefs of patients concerning transfusion.

(B) If the patient has a need for a transfusion.

(C) If the patient has a good intravenous line in place.

(D) If the patient is sleeping.

(131) As part of a blood transfusion lecture, you provide a scenario in which a patient experienced a severe reaction following a transfusion. Concerning ABO incompatibility, which of the following is correct?

(A) It is a form of hemoplastic blood reaction.

(B) It occurs when blood group O is transfused to blood group A.

(C) It is a hemolytic blood reaction.

(D) An agglutination reaction occurs.

(132) During an emergency simulation exercise, you present a scenario where a patient is having a severe blood transfusion reaction. Which of the following treatments would be the most useful in this scenario?

(A) Blood.

(B) Supplemental oxygen.

(C) Corticosteroids.

(D) Antihistamines.

(133) In a clinical skills lab, you teach nursing students about pre-transfusion safety checks. You ask which of the steps is not essential before commencing a blood transfusion. What is the correct answer?

(A) Check the blood donation date.

(B) Check the blood bag details.

(C) Check pre-transfusion vital signs.

(D) Check pre-transfusion blood glucose levels.

(134) As part of a teaching session on intravenous access, you provide a case study of a patient needing a peripheral line. You ask the students about the best location to place this line. Which of the following is correct?

(A) They are best placed in the large veins of the lower limbs.

(B) They are best placed on the hand veins.

(C) They are best placed on the dominant forearm.

(D) They are best placed on the nondominant forearm.

(135) You're teaching a class on venous access and its potential complications. Which of the following statements about venous access is correct?

(A) Central lines should be changed every five days.

(B) Peripheral lines are better for quick emergencies.

(C) Nurses do not need to worry about infections.

(D) Phlebitis is very uncommon with chemotherapy administration through IV lines.

(136) What is the primary purpose of the surgical time-out process?

(A) To ensure that the correct surgery is performed on the correct patient and the correct site.

(B) To confirm the patient's identity.

(C) To verify the type of anesthesia to be used.

(D) To finalize the surgical plan.

(137) You're discussing the importance of accuracy in pharmacological measures with a group of nurses. Why is accuracy vital in these measures?

(A) It affects the cost of medication.

(B) It affects the nurse's workload.

(C) It affects the patient's treatment.

(D) It affects the nurse's job performance.

(138) In a training session focused on drug dose calculation and administration, you ask your trainees why accuracy is critically important in these tasks. Which of the following is correct?

(A) Accuracy can affect the patient's treatment.

(B) Accuracy can save time for the nurse.

(C) Accuracy is a requirement for nurses' job satisfaction.

(D) Accuracy is not important in pharmacological measures.

(139) You're tutoring a group of nursing students about the routes of drug administration and bioavailability. Which route of drug administration has 100% bioavailability?

(A) Oral route.

(B) Intravenous route.

(C) Transdermal route.

(D) Inhalation route.

(140) In a lecture about nutritional support therapies, you ask your nursing students to identify the other term for total parenteral nutrition. Which of the following is correct?

(A) Hyperalimentation.

(B) Enteral nutrition.

(C) Intravenous infusion.

(D) Oral feeding.

(141) You're in the middle of a lecture about total parenteral nutrition. You provide a case scenario where a patient is unable to consume adequate nutrients through their digestive system. How are necessary nutrients such as minerals, electrolytes, vitamins, amino acids, and trace elements supplied in this case?

(A) Via the hyperalimentation catheter.

(B) Orally.

(C) Intramuscularly.

(D) Through the nose.

(142) During a clinical skills lab, you introduce a manikin patient who needs total parenteral nutrition. What is the recommended route for administering this treatment?

(A) Peripheral vein.

(B) Oral route.

(C) Central vein.

(D) Intramuscular route.

(143) In a pharmacology class, you present a scenario of a patient who has undergone surgery and is experiencing significant pain. What determines the dosage and strength for this patient's pain medication?

(A) The patient's age and gender.

(B) The patient's medical history.

(C) The patient's weight and height.

(D) The level of pain and type of pain.

(144) You're discussing pain management with your nursing students. Which of these are examples of non-opioid analgesics?

(A) Morphine and oxycodone.

(B) Aspirin and acetaminophen.

(C) Fentanyl and codeine.

(D) Methadone and hydromorphone.

(145) You’re discussing a patient who prefers nonpharmacological pain management techniques during a case study review. What are some examples of these techniques?

(A) Heat therapy, cold therapy, and massage.

(B) Antibiotics, corticosteroids, and diuretics.

(C) Chemotherapy, radiation therapy, and surgery.

(D) Cardiac catheterization, angioplasty, and bypass surgery.

(146) You present a scenario where a patient with dementia is showing signs of discomfort. What should healthcare providers do when assessing pain in patients who have difficulty communicating?

(A) Disregard their pain.

(B) Assume they have no pain.

(C) Use pain scales and observation.

(D) Rely solely on patient self-reports.

(147) During a lecture on pain management, you present a case where a patient has chronic pain and is involved in their treatment plan. What is the role of patient education in this case?

(A) To discourage patients from seeking pain relief.

(B) To promote self-management and adherence to the pain management plan.

(C) To minimize patient involvement in pain management.

(D) To discourage communication about pain with healthcare providers.

(148) You're explaining to your students the best practices in intravenous therapy. What is the rationale for using upper limbs for this therapy?

(A) Lower-limb phlebitis can be avoided.

(B) Upper limbs have larger veins.

(C) It is easier to access veins in upper limbs.

(D) Upper limbs are less prone to infections.

(149) During a skills lab session, you pose a question about who is authorized to care for central lines and venous access devices in intravenous therapy. Which of the following is correct?

(A) Physician.

(B) Nursing assistant.

(C) RN.

(D) Physical therapist.

(150) In a pharmacology lecture, you discuss a case where a nurse needs to clarify a patient's medications. What are reliable sources for the nurse to obtain information about this patient's medications?

(A) Patient's family members.

(B) Social media.

(C) Nurse's intuition.

(D) Nurse's drug handbook, nursing textbook, formulary, pharmacist, and trustworthy internet resources.

Test 2: Answers and Explanations

(1) (B) Uniform Anatomical Gift Act.

This act allows living clients to donate their body parts in the US. It allows relatives of a deceased individual to decide to donate an organ if the individual did not decide while alive. It also includes several regulations that prevent the sale or trafficking of human body parts.

(2) (A) Value history.

This document describes the beliefs, opinions, and principles of the client. Although it is not a legal document, it is useful in determining some decisions on how a patient is handled and how the beliefs that they hold affect their treatment and care.

(3) (A) Ask her to turn the stroke patient.

Turning the stroke patient does not require high professional judgment because the patient is stable. But resuscitating the 25-year-old man will require a general assessment of his condition, fluid status, and mental health status, which would be more appropriate for an RN to do.

(4) (D) None of the above.

Nursing case management involves developing, implementing, and evaluating patient health care plans. But beyond all of this, it is an effective method of delivering nursing care. It typically involves managing and coordinating care, identifying and effectively using resources, planning referrals, and connecting clients to services based on need.

(5) (D) All of the above.

The plan developed for each patient must be individualized based on the patient's condition and need. The plan must consider several factors about the client, such as the diagnosis, ability to take care of oneself, the currently prescribed treatment, and actual and potential problems. The plan must always remain up to date based on the current needs of the client.

(6) (B) HIPAA.

HIPAA protects the client's personal information (e.g., the name, date of birth, social security number, diagnosis, and treatment). This act ensures that only those involved in the management or care of the patient have access to health information.

(7) (C) Provide inaccurate information about their health status.

Client responsibilities include treating health care workers with respect, paying medical bills and resolving other financial obligations as soon as possible, reporting changes that are unexpected in their condition to health care professionals, providing accurate information about their health, following rules and regulations given upon admission, and being responsible for their behavior.

(8) (D) Rejection or acceptance of interventions on behalf of the patient.

The goal of advocacy is to speak on behalf of patients and defend their rights and interests at all times. Advocacy can be in different forms. It may involve extensive education and sensitization of the patient and client families. It also involves explaining diagnoses, tests or examination findings. However, it is not the place of the nurse to accept or reject an intervention on behalf of a patient. Let patients and their families decide what they want.

(9) (C) Assess the client.

The first step is to assess the client's needs and whether the nursing staff and other health care professionals can adequately meet the need.

(10) (D) All of the above.

To triage effectively, a nurse must be organized and composed. A nurse must be able to diagnose conditions appropriately and have a high suspicion index. A nurse must be an excellent time manager to ensure that the right medications are given at the right time in the right doses. Any RN must also be an expert manager of people to get them to work together as a team to achieve quality health care delivery.

(11) (D) All of the above.

A nurse should be able to communicate effectively with others so that work is done at the right time. A nurse should also plan work systematically, making room for changes in the status or condition of clients and priorities. The health care setting is usually very busy, and if care is not taken, less urgent tasks can get in the way of urgent tasks. Therefore, it is the responsibility of a nurse to decline such tasks when there are other urgent tasks to perform.

(12) (B) Sentinel event.

A sentinel event refers to an incident or accident that could potentially cause harm to a client. In this question, the sentinel event was the transfusion of the two pints of blood, which led to a severe transfusion reaction.

(13) (B) Outcome measures.

Outcome measures focus on the outcomes of care. They focus on the results that are obtained as a result of health care delivered to a client. They include MRSA infection rates, lengths of stay, the effectiveness of fall prevention, and morbidity rates.

(14) (D) All of the above.

Nurses collaborate with other members of the health care team to deliver quality health care. Nurses must maintain high professionalism, good interpersonal and communication skills, and sound judgment when interacting with other health care professionals.

(15) (D) All of the above.

Nurses can serve as patient advocates at interdisciplinary conferences, raising issues pertinent to client care. They can also resolve potential conflict issues and areas of misunderstanding with other professionals. Interdisciplinary conferences are necessary for the holistic management of patients. They provide the opportunity to contribute to client care, and learn and observe from the perspective of other health care professionals.

(16) (D) Frustration.

At this point, the people involved in the conflict feel like their needs, whatever they are, are being sidelined. It might be a need for respect, consideration of working hours, a bonus or raise, or a client feeling neglected.

(17) (B) Individuals responding to the frustrations and conclusions they have arrived at.

The action state of conflict is when individuals act on the frustrations and conclusions they have come to. At this point, the action taken differs. For some, the action taken may be lashing out in anger or physical assault. Others may withdraw and avoid the person involved.

(18) (A) Random blood glucose test.

The most important investigation for this client is a random blood glucose check because he is a known Type I DM. He is most likely suffering from hypoglycemia secondary to insulin overdose or administration without eating. Fasting blood glucose, urine tests, and CBC can also be useful later on. But at the moment, the most important test is random blood glucose.

(19) (C) As often as needed.

Health care plans should be revised as often as needed whenever there is a change in a patient's condition. Patients are always in a dynamic state. The plan of care must be adjusted to their needs. When there is an improvement, the plan of care should be updated; otherwise, the plan of care should be adjusted to suit the new state.

(20) (B) Ethical dilemmas cannot be avoided in nursing care.

As nurses practice the delivery of care, ethical dilemmas will definitely arise because there are different types of patients, conditions, and cases that will be encountered. The nurse must be grounded in the ethics of the profession to make the right decisions.

(21) (D) Both A and B.

The purpose of the code of ethics is to provide a framework for decision-making and to set responsibility reminders for nurses.

(22) (B) Revise the code of ethics.

The code of ethics is revised from time to time to cover development in the world. This includes changes in technology, the community, expanding nursing practice into advanced practice roles, research, education, health policy, and administration.

(23) (D) IV acetaminophen 900 mg STAT given. The patient reports pain as 5/10.

The right way to input information is the date, time, the drug and the correct route of administration, the dose, the frequency, and the assessment of the patient.

(24) (B) "I am sorry, I cannot allow you to see that."

Let her know that you must keep such information private. HIPAA protects the client's personal information (e.g., the name, date of birth, social security number, diagnosis, and treatment). This act ensures that only those involved in the management or care of the patient have access to health care information.

(25) (D) "I will get you a copy from the records office."

According to the patient's bill of rights, patients have the right to review their medical records and request an amendment of any inaccurate information.

(26) (B) It means: give medication 4 times daily.

PRN means as often as needed. Three times daily is TDS, and BD is twice daily. Drugs are usually administered as regularly as needed or as prescribed. “QDS” or “qid” is an abbreviation for the Latin term “quater in die”, which translates to “four times a day”.

(27) (D) Not evaluating the patient for stroke is negligence.

A transient ischemic attack is a risk factor for stroke, and not evaluating a TIA patient for stroke would be considered negligence.

(28) (C) A five-year-old boy whose weight for his age is below normal.

This child might need a targeted nutritional assessment because his weight for his age is already below normal. Target screening can be done when some people show strong tendencies, signs, or symptoms of a particular condition or disease. This target screening is also done when a client is at risk of a certain ailment or there is a need to rule out a possible condition.

(29) (A) Nonjudgmental behavior.

Nurses should be open, trusting, and nonjudgmental. No matter the condition, they should be open to understanding the client’s perspective, even if what the person is saying is not correct from a professional stance.

(30) (D) Exercise.

High-risk behaviors are actions that significantly increase the likelihood of harm, disease, or death. Most of these behaviors are modifiable behaviors that are based on choice. They can include diet, a sedentary lifestyle, violence, and drug abuse.

(31) (D) 4.

Physical readiness involves the measure of ability, the complexity of the task, the effect of the environment, the health status of the individual, and even gender. Mental readiness deals more with the cognitive and psychological aspects of readiness. Experiential readiness deals with the levels of aspiration, coping mechanisms used in the past, the locus of control orientation, and self-efficacy. Knowledge readiness refers to the current level of knowledge of the learner, the level of capacity to learn, and the preferred style of learning of the individual.

(32) (A) Avoid drinking or eating anything for eight hours before surgery.

Patients are generally advised to fast (nothing by mouth) for eight hours prior to surgery to prevent aspiration of gastric contents during anesthesia.

(33) (B) Moderately distressed, needs moderate resuscitation.

Each parameter in the APGAR score is assessed as 0, 1, or 2, and the total is added up to 10. If a child scored less than 4, then the child is in severe distress and will need urgent intensive care and resuscitation. A score of 4–6 is moderately distressed and requires moderate attention and resuscitation. Neonates who score 7 and above are in excellent condition.

(34) (D) Master toilet training.

Toddlers are at Erikson's second stage of development, called "autonomy vs. shame and doubt." At this stage, children are focused on the development of self-control. At this stage, they are expected to master toilet training.

(35) (B) Decreased self-consciousness.

WHO defines adolescence as between 10–19 years. There is increased identity definition at this stage of development. At this stage, you should expect to see attraction toward the opposite sex, increased self-consciousness, and seeking peer group acceptance.

(36) (D) Both A and B.

This is the final stage of psychosocial development and it is seen in the elderly. It is called the "integrity vs. despair" stage, and people at this point usually look retrospectively at the influence of the choices they made earlier in life. They experience a gradual decline in physical function and musculature, along with some of the changes that are associated with aging in their body systems.

(37) (D) Placenta separation.

Active management of the third stage of labor involves administering 10 IU of oxytocin a minute after delivery to help the uterus contract, ensuring that the entire placenta is delivered through controlled cord traction and uterine massage. Placenta separation occurs on its own, and only after it has occurred can the placenta be delivered through controlled cord traction.

(38) (B) A fetal heart Doppler.

The fetal heart Doppler is a device that is used to monitor the heartbeat of the fetus in the uterus. Using this device creates a simulation of the fetal heartbeat; some devices display the value per minute. The sounds can also be heard and counted over a minute.

(39) (D) An elevated fetal heart rate.

An elevated fetal heart rate can be a strong indicator of fetal distress. Heart rates exceeding 160 bpm are considered elevated and demand urgent medical attention. Decreased fetal movement is more useful before labor and is usually assessed through a fetal kick chart.

(40) (B) Postpartum hemorrhage.

Postpartum hemorrhage is defined as blood loss greater than 500 mL for SVD or greater than 1,000 mL after a cesarean section. It is also defined as any volume of blood loss that results in hemodynamic instability of the patient after delivery.

(41) (C) Comfort and safety.

The client care environment refers to the physical and social setting in which nursing care is provided. Assessing the client care environment involves considering factors such as safety, comfort, privacy, and cultural sensitivity. Safety is a priority, and nurses should ensure that environments where patients are to be attended to are continually kept safe from threats and potential hazards.

(42) (C) Deep vein thrombosis (DVT).

Swelling, warmth, and pain in a lower extremity can be signs of a deep vein thrombosis, a serious complication that can occur after surgery. The nurse should alert the healthcare provider immediately.

(43) (D) All of the above.

Some things that can be done to promote staff safety include providing education and training, providing PPE, creating a safe and ideal work environment, and encouraging staff communication.

(44) (B) Every two hours.

Patients who cannot change their positions by themselves should be turned every two hours while being kept in a position that will cause no harm and bring minimal stress to muscle groups. This should be done to prevent the formation of bed sores.

(45) (D) A patient who cannot communicate in English.

A patient who needs help communicating in English or the official language of communication in the client care environment is highly prone to identification errors. To avoid this, such patients have a right to an interpreter so they can understand all that is communicated to them.

(46) (C) Irrespective of where they occur and who is affected.

RNs should be trained to handle all kinds of emergencies, including those within or outside their medical facilities' confines and those within or outside their communities. Nurses' response to the crisis is not based on who is affected, nor is it based on color, race, or any other form of bias.

(47) (B) Ambulatory clients.

Ambulatory clients who require little or no assistance should be the first to be discharged after they have been treated, given prescriptions, and received other necessary instructions. Unstable patients are high-priority clients and are, therefore, not candidates for discharge.

(48) (A) It prevents sabotage and further risks to those affected.

RNs should be able to use intuition to discern and plan ahead for the most effective ways to communicate during emergencies. This will avoid sabotage and additional risks that can come to patients due to leaked information.

(49) (C) Nonbiological material that poses some form of harm to living beings.

Hazardous materials are defined as nonbiological materials that pose some form of harm to human beings, animals, and other living components of the environment. Hazardous materials can be anything, ranging from harmful chemicals and radiation to soiled and used equipment such as needles, which could become potential sources of infection.

(50) (A) Time, distance, and shielding.

Nurses and technicians should ensure clients have the most minimal exposure to radiation by minimizing exposure time, ensuring safe distance, and using proper shielding.

(51) (D) All of the above.

Nurses, alongside other health care staff, work together to assess clients' homes, identify safety concerns, offer solutions or modifications, and educate on safety issues to provide an enabling home environment for clients.

(52) (B) Slip-proof floors.

Slip-proof floors are crucial for improving the well-being of patients and adjusting their lifestyles to new health conditions. Slip-proof floors ensure that the patients will not be involved in accidents due to sudden slipping.

(53) (A) With labeling that provides specific information for identifying the nature of each hazardous material.

Hazardous materials should be properly labeled so that even the layman can identify the risk. There should, however, also be labeling that provides specific information for identifying the nature of each hazardous material.

(54) (B) The supervising or charge nurse and the risk management department.

Reports should go to the health care facility's supervising or charge nurse and the risk management department.

(55) (B) It prevents hazards, client complications, and injuries.

Inspecting equipment before use is crucial for preventing hazards, client complications, and injuries to health care workers and patients.

(56) (C) Report and remove the equipment from the client care area.

Unsafe and malfunctioning equipment should be reported and moved from the client care area to ensure optimal safety. Faulty equipment should only be discarded if it has been designated irredeemable by a professional technician.

(57) (C) These are control measures used to prevent the spread of infection among clients, whether or not they've been diagnosed with any infection.

Standard precautions are the minimum infection prevention practices that should be used in health care settings for all patients. They are designed to reduce the risk of transmission of microorganisms from recognized and unrecognized infection sources.

(58) (B) Proper hand hygiene.

Proper hand hygiene, such as washing with mild soap and water, disinfecting when necessary and wearing protective gloves, prevents thousands of infections from spreading in health care environments.

(59) (D) All of the above.

Only sterile items should be placed on the sterile field. Nurses should never have a sterile field below the waist level. They should not lean over or ever turn their backs to the sterile field. Coughing or sneezing over the sterile field contaminates it. All staff in or around a sterile field should wear gowns and gloves. Those working directly on the sterile field should use sterile masks.

(60) (A) It ensures that the technique is in line with generally accepted procedures.

RNs should evaluate and monitor the staff members when carrying out aseptic techniques to ascertain competency and adherence to procedures.

(61) (A) Higher respiratory rate.

A one-year-old baby has a smaller lung volume compared to an adult and therefore has to breathe faster to exchange gases. Babies also metabolize faster, so they need to exchange waste products faster than adults.

(62) (C) Depressed respiration.

Some of the other signs of opioid intoxication include euphoria, reduced anxiety, hypotension from hypovolemia, miosis, and altered regulation of body temperature.

(63) (B) Consent is not really needed for noninvasive procedures.

The testing kits and equipment should be by the patient's bedside to start any diagnostic test. The nurse should do a brief introduction of the whole process. The patient must give consent to the test before proceeding. Proper handwashing before and after the test is essential to keep the process aseptic.

(64) (B) Hemostasis.

You press the puncture site with sterile gauze until the blood stops flowing. Applying pressure in this way reduces the flow of blood to that vessel and also allows for clotting factors to quickly get to work.

(65) (A) Superficial vein.

Blood collection is from a superficial vein, usually in the upper limb. This is because superficial veins are close to the skin and are easily accessible.

(66) (D) All of the above.

The nurse should first explain the process to the patient and obtain consent. Then the nurse can gather materials. The skin is cleaned with an alcohol swab, and the arm is tied with a tourniquet to make the veins more visible. A cannula is slowly introduced into the vein, and blood is collected into a bottle.

(67) (D) None of the above.

Proteins, blood cells, glucose, and other chemicals are assayed in the urine. Urine is routinely collected for urinary tract infections, sexually transmitted infections, and renal diseases.

(68) (A) Esophageal.

Patients exposed to cigarette smoke are at risk of lung, esophageal, and oral cancers. Patients with a family history of cancer are at risk. Patients whose occupation exposes them to ultraviolet radiation are predisposed to skin cancers.

(69) (A) Back pain.

The major alterations that happen secondary to chemotherapy include weight changes, nausea and vomiting, mouth sores, anemia, sleep difficulty, skin and nail changes, loss of appetite, easy bruising and bleeding, and infections.

(70) (C) Infections, bleeding.

Some noninvasive procedures are costlier than invasive procedures. However, invasive procedures always have concerns around infections because the skin barrier is breached and bleeding. Once infections and bleeding are not present, recovery is usually swift.

(71) (A) Obtain informed consent.

Consent must always be obtained before beginning any procedure.

(72) (C) Central and peripheral.

There are two ways to secure intravenous access—central and peripheral access. A peripheral intravenous line is used for short-term purposes such as administering fluids, chemotherapy, and electrolytes. Central venous access is for more long-term purposes.

(73) (D) The patient should be in the prone position for catheter insertion.

This is false. To insert a urinary catheter, the patient should be in the supine position for insertion. The nurse should expose the patient's thighs and pelvic region. The patient separates the thighs to give access to the perineal area. The catheter is inserted into the urethral meatus and advanced above the point when urine is seen in the catheter. The nurse should inflate the catheter to secure it in the urethra. The catheter is then connected to the urine bag and attached to the patient's leg.

(74) (D) Muscle length.

Assessing the neurological system requires appropriately assessing the cranial nerves, level of consciousness, muscle tone, and mental status. A patient's level of consciousness is set as oriented to time, place, and person. A patient isn't fully conscious if he or she doesn't know the time of the day, is confused about the date, and doesn't know where he or she is.

(75) (B) Inability to make facial expressions.

The facial nerve is assessed for the ability to feel sensory impulses of the face and move the muscles of the face to make facial expressions.

(76) (D) None of the above.

Hyperglycemia can present with polydipsia, urinary frequency, blurred vision, dehydration, and fatigue.

(77) (D) All of the above.

General anesthesia makes the client completely unconscious. Patients are intubated and placed on mechanical ventilation throughout the procedure. It is laborious and requires continuous monitoring. It is also essential to monitor the amount of anesthetic given as it can have dangerous side effects.

(78) (A) L3/L4 vertebrae.

In spinal anesthesia, where an anesthetic is injected into the subarachnoid space, the sites for administration are either between the L3/L4 or the L4/L5 vertebrae.

(79) (A) Vasodilation.

In hypothermia, the body's temperature falls lower than normal, and the body tries to generate heat by shivering and conserve heat by vasoconstriction, *not* vasodilation.

(80) (B) Cover the baby's eyes.

The baby's eyes must be covered to prevent possible retinal damage. However, the baby cannot be fully clothed during phototherapy with lights, or the radiation will not penetrate the skin. The light should be close to the baby's skin, typically about 10 cm or as stated by the manufacturer.

(81) (C) Request an opportunity to perform an invasive procedure.

Physicians and licensed practitioners do most invasive procedures. But nurses can assist them, so it is necessary to know about these procedures, the steps, and the complications. Some invasive procedures include central venous lines, needle biopsies, spinal taps, and intubations.

(82) (B) Oxygen toxicity.

Oxygen toxicity is another complication to look out for. The blood is being saturated continually by air containing oxygen under high pressure. Thus, there is a tendency for the blood to be oversaturated with oxygen.

(83) (A) To maintain the airways.

Oxygen is administered before suctioning to maintain the airways during suctioning. Preoxygenation involves increasing inspired oxygen just before suctioning. It has been suggested that preoxygenation can prevent some of the side effects of endotracheal suctioning (for instance, hypoxemia).

(84) (D) All of the above.

The wound area is inspected regularly. The color, size, presence of pus, surrounding structures, and odor of the pus are examined. The drainage of the wound can be bloody, serous, serosanguinous, and purulent.

(85) (A) Post-dural puncture headache (PDPH).

Patients with spinal or epidural anesthesia should not raise their heads for a few hours after the procedure to prevent postdural puncture headaches (PDPHs). PDPH occurs as a result of the leakage of cerebrospinal fluid through the hole created by the needle when anesthesia is administered. The reduction in CSF volume causes a stretch of the cranial nerves, which presents as a headache. The headache is usually positional and frontal.

(86) (B) Place the patient prone with the head of the bed elevated at 45 degrees.

The patient is prone and the bed is elevated to a 45-degree position. This drains respiratory secretions from the posterior bronchus.

(87) (D) All of the above.

The surgical wound site is examined as part of care for ostomies. Nurses maintain the tubes' patency and change them as needed. For tracheostomies, the nurse monitors the input and output of respiratory secretions.

(88) (C) It is a connection between an artery and a vein.

An AV is a connection between an artery and a vein. "Arterio" refers to arteries; "venous" refers to veins.

(89) (C) Three months before dialysis.

An AV is a connection between an artery and a vein. It is done three months before the dialysis to allow for maturity.

(90) (A) Potassium (K).

Potassium (K) is the most abundant intracellular electrolyte. Sodium (Na) is the most abundant extracellular electrolyte. Calcium (Ca) is both intracellular and extracellular, but predominantly intracellular. Phosphorus (P) is mostly deposited in the bone, but also has some intracellular and extracellular qualities.

(91) (D) Hypokalemia.

Hypokalemia is the reduction in the potassium levels in the blood below the usual standard. Hypokalemia can be a result of diarrhea, vomiting, and diaphoresis. Hypokalemia is characterized by muscle weakness, tingling, numbness, constipation, and even cardiac arrest.

(92) (C) Diabetes insipidus.

In diabetes insipidus, there is a loss of large volumes of water, which results in a depleted fluid volume and an increase in osmotic concentration. Such can result in hypernatremia.

(93) (A) Bleeding from trauma.

Hypovolemia is a reduction in blood fluid. Hypovolemia may occur as a result of bleeding, vomiting, and diarrhea, but the most common cause is bleeding from trauma. Fluid overload does not cause hypovolemia. Gluttony only results in hypovolemia if there is associated vomiting and diarrhea, which is very severe.

(94) (D) None of the above.

Hemodynamics is the study of how blood generally flows through the blood vessels.

(95) (D) All of the above.

Nurses should know the complications, such as infections, trauma, hematomas, and scar tissue formation. Nurses should monitor the hemodynamic status of patients with arterial lines. They should also anticipate the complications and manage accordingly.

(96) (D) Give anticoagulant medications.

For a patient with a pacemaker, the insertion site of the pacemaker should be assessed for bleeding and infections. The nurse should maintain bed rest and avoid giving the patient heparin or aspirin, which are anticoagulants.

(97) (C) Only the telemetry technician should monitor the ECG.

Telemetry involves continuously monitoring and recording ECG strips. Telemetry is mostly done by a telemetry technician, but nurses can monitor telemetry too.

(98) (D) Chest X-ray.

Patients with impaired ventilation or oxygenation should be assessed with pulmonary function tests such as pulse oximetry, spirometry, lung compliance, and forced vital capacity. A chest X-ray, however, is not a pulmonary function test, even though it can be used to visualize the lungs and pleural space.

(99) (C) It does not include the financial implications of the treatment.

This is false. As part of the treatment plan, the patient should be told about the treatment procedures and the financial cost of each treatment. Nurses should teach patients about home care strategies for their illnesses. The patients should receive a follow-up schedule as part of the treatment plan.

(100) (B) Counsel the patient and allay his fears.

The best next course of action is to counsel and allay the patient's fear, as excessive and frequent urination is a known side effect of medications used to treat heart failure and hypertensive heart disease.

(101) (A) Colostomy.

A colostomy is a surgical procedure done to establish an artificial connection between the lumen of the colon and the skin, which has varying indications. The indication in this case is to rest the repair site of the perforated bowel. It is important to be aware of common surgical procedures, indications, and effects on management.

(102) (A) Speech difficulty.

Speech difficulty is not a primary issue related to mobility. It is, however, related to the primary pathology. Other answer options are systemic complications of prolonged immobility and should be anticipated and prevented.

(103) (B) III, I, IV, II.

Based on the WHO analgesic ladder, pain management is usually started with the least non-opioids to opioids and, finally, other interventional treatments to manage severe pain.

(104) (C) Knee.

Pressure sores commonly occur on bony prominences, which are in prolonged contact with the bed. Due to immobility, patients usually lie decubitus in bed; thus, the knees are usually facing upward and are rarely in contact with the bed.

(105) (B) Patient feels refreshed after waking up.

Feeling refreshed after waking up is the best response to assess the quality of sleep, as the duration of sleep and other parameters do not fully reflect improvement in insomnia management.

(106) (B) Vitamin E deficiency.

Vitamin E deficiency is not closely related to delayed wound healing. Deficiencies in Vitamin C, A, zinc, copper, and low serum protein are associated with poor wound healing postoperatively as they are required for collagen formation.

(107) (D) Poor tissue perfusion.

Poor tissue perfusion is an intrinsic factor related to pressure sores. Adequate oxygenation prevents pressure sores. Elevated blood pressure has little effect on pressure sores. Poor turning in bed is an extrinsic factor related to pressure sores.

(108) (A) A central venous catheter.

A central venous catheter is the best route for administration of TPN as it lasts longer, it does not get blocked easily, and nutrients enter the bloodstream faster, unlike the other routes.

(109) (C) 2.

Muscle power is graded on a scale of 0 to 5.

0 – No movement at all.
1 – Flicker of movement.
2 – Cannot move against gravity but can move from side to side.

3 – Can move against gravity but not with resistance.
4 – Can move against gravity and with mild to moderate resistance.
5 – Full power.

(110) (A) Limited physical examination.

During a detailed health assessment of a patient, a complete physical examination should be done rather than a limited physical examination.

(111) (D) Bereavement.

The Kübler-Ross model of grief includes the following stages: Denial is when the person refuses to accept the loss that has occurred. Anger can be directed at oneself, the family, friends, or the world. Bargaining involves bargaining with a higher power. Depression is felt when the person begins to really feel the loss. Acceptance is living with the new reality that the loved one is truly gone. Bereavement is not a component of the model.

(112) (B) A neurosurgeon.

A neurosurgeon is not necessarily needed in the management of cerebral palsy. Professionals needed include a pediatric neurologist, pediatric nurse, occupational therapist, physiotherapist, nutritionist, speech therapist, ENT surgeon, and orthopedic surgeon.

(113) (A) High steppage gait.

High steppage gait is usually seen in patients with sciatic nerve injury, causing foot drop, and hence the need for high leg clearance during walking. Waddling gait is seen in developmental dysplasia of the hip. Antalgic is seen in pain of limb infection, and Festinant gait is usually seen in Parkinson's disease.

(114) (B) Drug-seeking behavior.

Ray is exhibiting drug-seeking behavior. Other manifestations of drug-seeking behavior include claiming medications have been exhausted, falsifying prescriptions, or always having an ailment that requires medication.

(115) (D) All of the above.

When clients are diagnosed, the nurse needs to observe them and their reactions. Some clients might be defensive, and others might feel ashamed. Some clients might immediately admit their problem and then seek a way out. Others might blame others and rationalize their behavior. Some clients might present with low self-esteem masked with a buoyant personality or aggression.

(116) (D) All of the above.

Sexual addiction is a non-substance–related addiction. For clients in this category, impulse control counseling and therapy would be useful. Cognitive-behavioral therapy and drug therapy can also be beneficial in addressing these disorders.

(117) (D) Assess for airway patency.

Upon emergence from anesthesia, the nurse's first priority is always to assess airway patency. Once this is established, other priorities can be attended to.

(118) (B) Tendency to inflict self-harm or harm others.

Some of the risk factors for self-harm and violence to others include a history of depression, a history of self-harm, a history of depression, age greater than 45 years, past suicide attempts, non-heterosexual orientations, and joblessness.

(119) (A) Quickly apologize and speak to the head.

Nurses must always ensure they allow for their clients' cultural practices and beliefs when providing care. This determines if the care will be received or rejected many times. No matter how different a culture might be, a nurse must respect it as long as it does not harm the client or other clients in the hospital.

(120) (D) Assessment of discipline techniques.

End-of-life care should be adequately provided for clients who need it. This care might include proper hygiene, ensuring the patient is comfortable, and providing privacy. It might include proper turning and positioning of the patient at regular intervals. It can also include massage, therapy, and any other treatment the client needs.

(121) (B) Laissez-faire.

Some families operate in an authoritarian structure where the leader makes all the decisions without room for deliberation among family members. Others run a democratic structure where all family members can deliberate on matters and decisions to be made. Some other families run a laissez-faire leadership where individuals within the family unit are left to make their own decisions while the leaders support and provide the needed resources.

(122) (A) Accepting the loss, coping, altering the environment, resuming a healthy life.

Worden's four tasks of mourning include accepting the loss, coping with the loss, altering the environment to cope with the loss, and resuming a healthy life.

(123) (A) Bipolar disorder.

Bipolar disorder presents with episodes of manic and hypomanic depression occurring at intervals. Signs and symptoms include elevated mood, irritability, depressed mood, restlessness, loss of inhibition, increased sexual drive, loss of sleep, and grandiose delusion.

(124) (B) Sitting for long hours.

Sitting for long hours at a stretch can be a risk factor for cardiovascular diseases. It can be an indication of a sedentary lifestyle, which is also a risk factor for cardiovascular illnesses and obesity. It can also lead to diabetes, increased cholesterol, DVT, and dementia.

(125) (D) Both A and B.

There is increased cardiac output in both stages for different reasons. In the alarm stage, these manifestations aim to prepare the patient to flee. The resistance stage is marked by increased cardiac output and a maintained respiratory rate and blood pressure increase. Here, the body is trying to deal with the effects of stress.

(126) (B) "Thank you so much for telling me about your wife. I am sure she is an amazing person. But can we also discuss your medications, so we can get you back home to be with her soon?"

This is called focusing. A nurse must be able to focus the discussion on the important issues at hand, even when the client wants to divert to other things not as important or pertinent at the moment.

(127) (A) Every human has an allergy.

It is not established that all human beings have allergies; however, signs and symptoms of allergic reactions may vary per person and per exposure. Some reactions can also be life-threatening.

(128) (D) Give both one hour apart and flush the line in between both doses.

This is the most appropriate way to give such a combination, as giving them in quick succession can cause a chemical reaction that can damage the vein or cause a reaction. This is why a good knowledge of chemistry and pharmacology is important in nursing practice to identify such issues.

(129) (D) None of the above.

Mixing any substance with blood during a transfusion is not advisable to prevent lysing blood components or causing a transfusion reaction. Even if the substance is not known to cause a reaction, it should not be mixed with blood.

(130) (D) If the patient is sleeping.

Instead of assessing if the patient is asleep, it is better to assess the vital signs and sensorium of the patient. The religious or cultural beliefs of patients are very important as some people with religious beliefs do not accept blood transfusions. One example is Jehovah's Witnesses.

(131) (C) It is a hemolytic blood reaction.

It is a hemolytic agglutination reaction that occurs due to the transfusion of mismatched blood types.

(132) (B) Supplemental oxygen.

There may be an imminent cardiorespiratory failure in severe blood transfusion reactions, and the patient may require supplemental oxygen and pharmaceuticals. Corticosteroids and antihistamines are useful in mild to moderate reactions. Blood is not needed for this emergency.

(133) (D) Check pre-transfusion blood glucose levels.

It is very important to check the blood donation date as this will help to know how fresh the blood is, as some conditions warrant fresh whole blood. Also, ensuring the blood bag details are correct will help prevent blood transfusion reactions due to clerical errors. Pre-transfusion vital signs help to know when the patient reacts to the blood. Blood glucose levels do not affect blood transfusion.

(134) (D) They are best placed on the nondominant forearm.

Peripheral venous catheters are best placed on the nondominant forearm to enable the patient to use the dominant limb for other activities. Lower extremities are avoided because of attendant complications of phlebitis.

(135) (B) Peripheral lines are better for quick emergencies.

Because of the level of expertise needed to secure central venous access, it is less suitable for emergencies. Central lines should be changed every 48 hours. Infections should be a concern with venous lines. Chemotherapy is notable for cellular damage.

(136) (A) To ensure that the correct surgery is performed on the correct patient and the correct site.

The primary purpose of the surgical time-out process is to ensure patient safety by confirming the correct patient, correct procedure, and correct surgical site.

(137) (C) It affects the patient's treatment.

Accuracy in dosage, routes, and concentration of medications is important to ensure proper patient treatment. If the dosage is less than what is needed, then the effect of the drug will not be as potent as it should be. If the dosage is higher, then toxicity might set in.

(138) (A) Accuracy can affect the patient's treatment.

Accuracy in pharmacological measures, such as medication dosage calculations, is critical to ensure that patients receive the correct amount of medication their health care provider prescribes. Incorrect dosages can have serious consequences, including ineffective treatment or adverse effects on the patient's health.

(139) (B) Intravenous route.

All the medication administered into the veins will reach the target organs; hence only the intravenous route has 100% bioavailability.

(140) (A) Hyperalimentation.

Total parenteral nutrition, known as hyperalimentation, is administered through a more prominent vein, such as the subclavian vein. Hyperalimentation can meet all dietary requirements, with feedings containing minerals, electrolytes, vitamins, amino acids, and trace elements supplied via the hyperalimentation catheter, which the physician surgically implants.

(141) (A) Via the hyperalimentation catheter.

Minerals, electrolytes, vitamins, amino acids, and trace elements are supplied via the hyperalimentation catheter, which is surgically implanted.

(142) (C) Central vein.

The recommended route for administering total parenteral nutrition is through the central vein. Parenteral nutrition cannot be given via peripheral veins because of the increased risk of thrombophlebitis when administered peripherally. The central line also allows a large quantity of nutrients to be given over a shorter period of time.

(143) (D) The level of pain and type of pain.

The level of pain and type of pain are what will determine the medication dosage and strength of the pain medication to be administered.

(144) (B) Aspirin and acetaminophen.

Aspirin and acetaminophen are examples of non-opioid analgesics. The rest of the options, morphine and oxycodone, fentanyl, codeine, methadone, and hydromorphone, are examples of opioid analgesics.

(145) (A) Heat therapy, cold therapy, and massage.

Heat therapy, cold therapy, and massage are examples of nonpharmacological pain management techniques.

(146) (C) Use pain scales and observation.

With the use of pain scales and observation, a subjective assessment can be made of the patient's pain level.

(147) (B) To promote self-management and adherence to the pain management plan.

Patient education promotes self-management and adherence to the pain management plan.

(148) (A) Lower-limb phlebitis can be avoided.

Upper limbs are used wherever possible to avoid lower-limb phlebitis and emboli. DVT is very common with lower limb veins, and it should be avoided at all costs. Upper limb veins can also sometimes be more accessible than lower limb veins. They are also easy for cannula placement and infusion drips.

(149) (C) RN.

RNs are responsible for caring for central lines and venous access devices in intravenous therapy.

(150) (D) Nurses' drug handbook, nursing textbook, formulary, pharmacist, and trustworthy internet resources.

The nurses' drug handbook, a nursing textbook, a formulary, a pharmacist, and trustworthy internet resources are reliable sources that nurses can access and obtain information about a patient's medications.

Test 3 Questions

(1) Greg was admitted to a hospital after an automobile accident in which he lost a lot of blood. His hematocrit was very low, and a transfusion was recommended. However, he declined to receive blood via transfusion for personal reasons. What did Greg exercise here?

(A) Right to privacy.

(B) Self-Determination Act.

(C) Health care proxy.

(D) Uniform Anatomical Gift Act.

(2) Which of the following is not true about delegation?

(A) It means the transfer of responsibility.

(B) The nurse delegating retains no responsibility for the outcome of the delegated task.

(C) The nurse delegating still retains responsibility for the outcome of the delegated task.

(D) All of the above.

(3) What is the basis when selecting the right person for a task?

(A) Skills and knowledge.

(B) Physical fitness.

(C) Nationality.

(D) Literacy.

(4) There are ______ types of healthcare reimbursement.

(A) 2.

(B) 3.

(C) 4.

(D) 5.

(5) What models are used for case management?

(A) Double case model.

(B) ProACT model.

(C) REACT model.

(D) All of the above.

(6) A patient who cannot speak or understand English enters the hospital. As a nurse, what is your next course of action?

(A) Find out what language the patient speaks and get an interpreter.

(B) Refer the patient based on language difference.

(C) Try to use signs to communicate.

(D) None of the above.

(7) Prior to a hysterectomy, a patient was properly counseled by a nurse on the implications, benefits, risks, side effects, and alternatives. Then the client signed a document that stated she fully understood everything explained to her. What was displayed here?

(A) Consent.

(B) Implied consent.

(C) Informed consent.

(D) All of the above.

(8) A nurse that is not present during ward rounds cannot be a good advocate for patients. This is because:

(A) Important decisions are made during the rounds.

(B) The rounds show the nurse's desire to be promoted.

(C) Rounds are meant to give a chance for exercise, and the nurse avoided extra exercise.

(D) The medical doctors will not be happy with the nurse for being absent during the rounds.

(9) What are some common referral resources?

(A) Social workers.

(B) Self-help.

(C) Shelters and housing.

(D) All of the above.

(10) What prioritization framework places physiological needs as a top priority?

(A) Resuscitation.

(B) Maslow's Hierarchy of Needs.

(C) Agency policies.

(D) All of the above.

(11) What areas benefit the most from performance improvement?

(A) Highest-risk areas.

(B) Lowest-risk areas.

(C) Lowest monetary areas.

(D) None of the above.

(12) What type of variance occurs when a part of the process is vulnerable to human error or is faulty?

(A) Random variance.

(B) Specific variance.

(C) Standard deviation.

(D) All of the above.

(13) What is currently the most popular performance improvement activity?

(A) PDCA cycle.

(B) Six Sigma method.

(C) Method de jour.

(D) None of the above.

(14) Which of the following are non-licensed?

(A) LPNs.

(B) RNs.

(C) Nursing assistants.

(D) None of the above.

(15) What specialty is primarily involved with a patient's functional abilities?

(A) Neurosurgeon.

(B) Gynecologist.

(C) Physical therapist.

(D) Occupational therapist.

(16) Two of your nursing staff were involved in a conflict during working hours. The options to resolve this conflict are not completely satisfactory to both parties. According to Lewin, what type of conflict is this?

(A) Avoidance-Avoidance.

(B) Avoidance-Acceptance.

(C) Approach-Avoidance.

(D) Double Approach-Avoidance.

(17) Some of the most common causes of conflict in the healthcare setting include:

(A) Disrespect.

(B) Overworking.

(C) Ill health.

(D) All of the above.

(18) Multiple injured patients are brought to the emergency room. A patient sustained a fracture, major lacerations, and bruises from an auto crash. What is your next line of action?

I – Inform doctors on call.

II – Get materials ready for suturing.

III – Administer ATS.

IV – Refer the patient.

(A) I, II, III

(B) I, II, IV

(C) I, III, II

(D) IV

(19) What should guide the delivery of healthcare?

(A) Pathophysiology.

(B) Physiology.

(C) Presentation.

(D) All of the above.

(20) A woman refuses immunization of her child for spiritual reasons. What should you do as a nurse?

(A) Counsel and educate her.

(B) Document her refusal.

(C) A and B.

(D) Immunize the child anyway.

(21) A nurse has the fundamental responsibility to:

(A) Alleviate suffering.

(B) Promote health.

(C) Prevent illness.

(D) All of the above.

(22) What is the right way to input information for clients?

(A) 09/10/20 1145 hrs. IV acetaminophen 900 mg stat given. Pain has subsided.

(B) 09/10/20 1145 hrs. IV acetaminophen 300 mg total dose given. Pain reported 2/10.

(C) 09/10/20 1145 hrs. IV acetaminophen given. The patient is feeling better.

(D) 09/10/20 1145 hrs. IV acetaminophen 300 mg STAT given. Patient reports pain as 2/10.

(23) You receive a call from one of your friends about her brother's wife, who has been admitted for two days. She wants to know what the diagnosis is. What should be your response?

(A) "Stop asking me these questions; it is against the law!"

(B) "I am sorry. I cannot give out such information about my clients."

(C) "What do you know about HIPAA?"

(D) Cut the call.

(24) A patient who only speaks Spanish enters the emergency room. You are the nurse on duty and speak Spanish but are not fluent. What should you do?

(A) Speak English and use signs to ask the patient to leave.

(B) Speak Spanish and reassure the patient that you will get an interpreter with a better command of the language.

(C) Interpret as much as you can and hope the client understands.

(D) Refer the patient.

(25) A woman visits the hospital with bruises and a black eye. You suspect physical abuse by her partner. She confides in you that this is true but asks you not to report it. What do you do?

(A) Follow her wishes.

(B) Document and report it.

(C) Scold the patient.

(D) Call her partner up to talk.

(26) Which of the following orders is most likely incorrect?

(A) IV acetaminophen 600 mg STAT for postoperative pain.

(B) IV morphine 150 mg STAT for postoperative pain.

(C) IV pentazocine 30 mg STAT for postoperative pain.

(D) B and C.

(27) A patient who has just suffered a stroke is brought into the emergency room. An urgent CT reveals a hemorrhagic stroke. What should be done next?

(A) Start medications.

(B) Look for relatives to sign the informed consent.

(C) Prepare for craniotomy.

(D) Admit the patient for bed rest.

(28) A 35-year-old woman presents with galactorrhea and has been unable to conceive. What targeted assessment would she benefit from?

(A) Complete blood count.

(B) Nutritional assessment.

(C) Hormonal profile.

(D) All of the above.

(29) Which of the following is false about high-risk behaviors?

(A) They are activities that increase the likelihood of harm.

(B) They are all modifiable.

(C) All risks are modifiable.

(D) None of the above.

(30) Which of the following is not a major determinant of health risks?

(A) Age.

(B) Socioeconomic status.

(C) Hobbies.

(D) None of the above.

(31) A patient with a motor impairment must learn to properly clean their wounds. What type of readiness to learn is most essential?

(A) Experiential readiness.

(B) Knowledge readiness.

(C) Physical readiness.

(D) All of the above.

(32) In which ways can nurses intervene in community health education?

(A) Oral presentations.

(B) Policy approval.

(C) Multidisciplinary cooperation.

(D) A and C.

(33) What is false about the New Ballard scale?

(A) It assesses physical and neuromuscular maturity.

(B) It is graded from 0 to 5.

(C) A scarf sign is a parameter.

(D) Heel-to-ear movement is a parameter.

(34) At what stage do disabilities that affect development become more obvious?

(A) Erikson's initiative vs. guilt stage.

(B) Erikson's industry vs. inferiority stage.

(C) Adolescence.

(D) Toddler.

(35) Which age group begins to form closer and stronger relationships with others?

(A) Young adults.

(B) Middle-aged adults.

(C) Elderly adults.

(D) All of the above.

(36) What musculoskeletal changes are observed among the elderly?

(A) Increased muscle mass.

(B) Increased intervertebral disc spaces.

(C) Reduced muscle tone and strength.

(D) B and C.

(37) What is the EDD of a woman with LMP on March 20, 2023?

(A) November 25, 2023.

(B) December 20, 2023.

(C) December 25, 2023.

(D) January 20, 2024.

(38) What parameters are used to monitor a newborn's growth and development?

(A) OFC.

(B) Length.

(C) Feeding.

(D) All of the above.

(39) How often should the umbilical cord be cleaned after birth?

(A) Every hour.

(B) Once every two days.

(C) Weekly.

(D) Several times a day.

(40) As a nurse, how can you ensure a woman can breastfeed her baby correctly?

(A) Educate her.

(B) Breastfeed for her.

(C) Demonstrate it and let her watch you, then let her do it herself.

(D) Make sure she talks about breastfeeding a lot.

(41) Which of the following best defines the client care environment?

(A) The physical and social setting in which nursing care is provided.

(B) The home environment of the client and the environment of the healthcare facility.

(C) The environment of the healthcare facility alone.

(D) The total of all the environments a client is exposed to.

(42) To ensure a safe client care environment, the nurse should do all of the following except:

(A) Ensure the environment is safe from threats and potential hazards.

(B) Assess the quality of the client's home environment.

(C) Regulate the environment to minimize falls and injuries.

(D) Assess for and eliminate factors that can trigger self-harm in clients.

(43) What is the best method to signal staff members about an unconscious patient's health state and safety in a private room?

(A) Bedside monitors.

(B) Call bell.

(C) An intercom system.

(D) Communication boards.

(44) Which of the following is false about patient positioning methods?

(A) Clients should be supported and made comfortable in the Sims position with pillows.

(B) The Sims position is halfway between the prone position and the lateral position.

(C) The Sims position is not the same as the semi-prone position.

(D) The Sims position is not the same as the prone position.

(45) What is the recommended minimum number of identifiers assigned to each client?

(A) 1.

(B) 2.

(C) 3.

(D) 4.

(46) Which of the following can be classified as an internal disaster?

(A) A bomb blast that has occurred within the community.

(B) A fire outbreak at a client's home.

(C) A loaded truck that brings victims of a massive hurricane from a community nearby.

(D) None of the above.

(47) The principles of triage require that:

(A) The most critical situations be attended to first.

(B) 10% of clients be discharged immediately if an emergency occurs.

(C) The fittest clients are recruited to assist with critical situations.

(D) All of the above.

(48) What is the right application of ergonomic principles in the healthcare environment?

(A) Use a specially designed wheelchair to transport a client with a lumbar spine injury.

(B) Help clients decide the right assistive device to use for their unique needs.

(C) Use tailored equipment to provide physiotherapy to individual clients.

(D) All of the above.

(49) Keep your feet apart when lifting an object because it will:

(A) Channel all your strength into lifting the weight properly.

(B) Provide a secure base for better balance.

(C) Ensure your feet are not in the way of the other persons who are lifting the weight with you.

(D) All of the above.

(50) Which client would be more prone to repetitive stress injury?

(A) A client who is currently undergoing physiotherapy.

(B) A client who mostly maintains the same position due to immobility or weakness in certain muscle groups.

(C) A client who has been placed on bed rest for three days.

(D) A client who exercises every day.

(51) Why is it important for nurses to consider client pathophysiology when proffering home safety solutions?

(A) To ensure clients have minimal exposure to radiation.

(B) To minimize exposure time.

(C) To provide clients with the right procedures to handle biohazardous materials.

(D) To ensure clients have an appropriate home environment for quick response and adjustment to new health challenges.

(52) Which of the following are biohazardous materials?

(A) Sharp tools.

(B) Used hospital beddings.

(C) Cleaning agents.

(D) Plastic wrappers.

(53) What information should be included in formal reports for incidents and other irregular occurrences?

(A) The names of healthcare workers who were contacted to attend the event.

(B) The date and time of the event.

(C) The place where the event occurred.

(D) All of the above.

(54) What are the different types of variances that should be recorded as irregular or out-of-place occurrences?

(A) Practitioner, system, and institutional.

(B) Patient, system, and institutional.

(C) Practitioner, system, and patient.

(D) None of the above.

(55) What are transmission-based precautions?

(A) Measures taken to prevent the transfer of disease-causing organisms from one person or object to another.

(B) Infection-control measures to prevent infection spread among clients, whether or not they've been diagnosed with any infection.

(C) Preventive and infection-control measures utilized to combat and inhibit the spread of specific infections.

(D) Specialized equipment used to protect specific body areas from injury and exposure to infectious agents.

(56) To educate clients and staff members on infection prevention and control measures:

(A) Evaluate the impact and effectiveness of such educational sessions.

(B) Assess the educational needs of these groups.

(C) Plan educational activities to meet the unique educational needs of these groups.

(D) All of the above.

(57) Which of the following is improper to do for immunocompromised clients who are susceptible to infection after exposure?

(A) Isolate them from other people until they have attained some level of recovery and immunity.

(B) Provide special care only when there is an infection outbreak.

(C) Utilize standard precautions when attending to them at all times.

(D) Protect them from infections that might not pose a threat to non-compromised clients.

(58) What should nurses do if they need to cough or sneeze when working on a sterile field?

(A) Turn their backs to the sterile field and cough or sneeze.

(B) Cover their nose and mouth with their hands.

(C) Move away from the sterile field before they cough or sneeze.

(D) Cough or sneeze over the sterile field since they have a nose mask on.

(59) In which situations may restraints and safety devices be required?

(A) To prevent infection in patients.

(B) To improve patient mobility.

(C) To prevent safety threats such as falls.

(D) To give patients a sense of autonomy.

(60) Which of the following is an inappropriate method of restraint?

(A) Belts and jackets that prevent limb movement.

(B) Physical restraint from a nurse.

(C) Medicine that keeps the patient immobile.

(D) Isolation in one room with no means of exit.

(61) Where would you check for the radial pulse?

(A) Lateral aspect of the arm.

(B) Medial aspect of the arm.

(C) Lateral aspect of the wrist.

(D) Medial aspect of the wrist.

(62) How much of the arm should be covered by the blood pressure cuff when checking for blood pressure?

(A) 1/2 of the upper arm.

(B) 2/3 of the upper arm.

(C) The entire arm.

(D) ¼ of the arm.

(63) What equipment must match for blood glucose testing?

(A) Strip and lancet.

(B) Meter and lancet.

(C) Strip and meter.

(D) All must match.

(64) ECG leads are routinely placed on all the following parts of the body except the:

(A) Chest.

(B) Hands.

(C) Legs.

(D) Head.

(65) Why do we use standardized values?

(A) For competition among labs.

(B) To compare with patient values.

(C) To maintain the same values across laboratories.

(D) All the above.

(66) Why do we use a tourniquet in venipuncture?

(A) To arrest blood flow.

(B) To engorge the veins.

(C) To make the veins visible.

(D) All of the above.

(67) Urine can be routinely collected to investigate all of the following except:

(A) Sexually transmitted infections.

(B) Renal diseases.

(C) Urinary tract infections.

(D) Respiratory tract infections.

(68) What is the role of a nurse to patients who are at risk?

(A) Identify them.

(B) Educate them.

(C) Refer them.

(D) A and B.

(69) A patient presents with skin cancer. Which of the following is not helpful to rule out causes and major risk factors?

(A) Occupation.

(B) Choice of diet.

(C) Family history of skin cancer.

(D) Personal history of skin cancer.

(70) What is the initial sign to look out for when a patient might be hemorrhaging?

(A) Hypotension.

(B) Hypertension.

(C) Fever.

(D) Pain.

(71) What position is used to pass the NG tube in a conscious patient?

(A) Trendelenburg's position.

(B) Left lateral decubitus position.

(C) High Fowler's position.

(D) Right lateral decubitus position.

(72) At what angle should the needle be placed into the vein in IV cannulations?

(A) 20–40 degrees.

(B) 10–20 degrees.

(C) 45–90 degrees.

(D) 15–30 degrees.

(73) Which of the following must always be done before the urine bag is emptied?

(A) Remove the catheter.

(B) Close the outlet.

(C) Note the volume of the urine.

(D) Pull the catheter to see if it's in place.

(74) Power in muscles is graded from:

(A) 1–5.

(B) 2–10.

(C) 0–5.

(D) -1–6.

(75) How many cranial nerves are present in the human body?

(A) 11.

(B) 10.

(C) 12.

(D) 20.

(76) Which of the following is false about therapeutic procedures?

(A) They're always medical.

(B) They can be surgical.

(C) They can be performed to remove foreign objects.

(D) They can be performed to repair wounds.

(77) What is the major role of the nurse in a surgical procedure?

(A) To help educate the patient.

(B) To help move the patient.

(C) To convince the patient.

(D) All of the above.

(78) Some diseases that are commonly transmitted by needle pricks include:

(A) Hepatitis B.

(B) Hepatitis A.

(C) Leukemia.

(D) All of the above.

(79) What are coping mechanisms?

(A) Thoughts, behaviors, and emotions.

(B) Physiological adaptations of the heart.

(C) Family patterns.

(D) All of the above.

(80) The most effective way to monitor bilirubin levels is to:

(A) Check skin color.

(B) Check stool color.

(C) Check eye color.

(D) Check blood levels in the lab.

(81) What are the types of needle biopsy?

(A) Fine needle aspiration and core needle biopsy.

(B) Liver and lung biopsy.

(C) Endoscopic biopsy and vacuum biopsy.

(D) All of the above.

(82) One basic technique to prevent infection in patients on a ventilator is:

(A) Antibiotics.

(B) Blood culture.

(C) Handwashing.

(D) All of the above.

(83) Which of the following statements is false?

(A) The tip of the suction catheter should be lubricated before advancing.

(B) Suctioning cannot be done more than once.

(C) Oxygen is given before suctioning.

(D) Only the nose can be suctioned.

(84) All of the following are examples of open wounds except:

(A) Abrasions.

(B) Punctures.

(C) Gunshot wounds.

(D) Hematomas.

(85) Patients who were under general anesthesia might feel exhausted and weak after they regain consciousness. What should the nurse do?

(A) Monitor vitals.

(B) Reassure the patient.

(C) Call the doctor for help.

(D) A and B.

(86) Postural drainage is most beneficial in all of the following conditions except:

(A) COPD.

(B) Bronchiectasis.

(C) Lung abscess.

(D) Acute rhinitis.

(87) What are two types of dialysis?

(A) Hemodialysis and serodialysis.

(B) Hemodialysis and perineal dialysis.

(C) Hemodialysis and peritoneal dialysis.

(D) Hemodialysis and renal transplant.

(88) What organ function does dialysis replace?

(A) The kidneys' ultrafiltration function.

(B) The liver's detoxification function.

(C) The kidneys' hemopoietic function.

(D) The kidneys' blood pressure regulation.

(89) What stage of renal failure is an indication for dialysis?

(A) Stage II.

(B) Stage III.

(C) Stage IV.

(D) Stage V.

(90) Which is the most abundant extracellular cation?

(A) Cl.

(B) Na.

(C) K.

(D) Mg.

(91) Which of the following is involved in neither muscular nor cardiac contractions?

(A) Na.

(B) K.

(C) Ca.

(D) None of the above.

(92) A patient is observed to be dyspneic, with edema of the lower and upper limbs. He is on an infusion of normal saline. His blood pressure is elevated. What is the first line of action?

(A) Stop the fluid infusion.

(B) Commence Lasix.

(C) Adjust the position.

(D) Reduce the fluid infusion.

(93) What is the first line of treatment in hypovolemia?

(A) Sutures.

(B) Resuscitation.

(C) Fluid restriction.

(D) None of the above.

(94) Arterial lines cannot be placed in the:

(A) Femoral artery.

(B) Brachial artery.

(C) Radial artery.

(D) Common interosseous artery.

(95) What are some of the complications of a pacemaker?

(A) Pneumothorax.

(B) Hemothorax.

(C) Cardiac tamponade.

(D) All of the above.

(96) Which of the following is easily done with the knowledge of the heart's electrical impulse?

(A) Interpretation of blood sugar values.

(B) Interpretation of ECG.

(C) Interpretation of EEG.

(D) All of the above.

(97) Patients should be given a good education on any disease condition they have. This information should include the disease's:

(A) Pathophysiology.

(B) Etiology.

(C) Signs and symptoms.

(D) All of the above.

(98) Why must nurses explain the signs and symptoms of a disease to clients?

(A) For prompt self-medication.

(B) For prompt presentation at the hospital as necessary.

(C) To educate others with a similar condition.

(D) B and C.

(99) Features of hypernatremia do not include:

(A) Thirst.

(B) Agitation.

(C) Restlessness and confusion.

(D) Arrhythmias.

(100) You are the nurse on duty in a ward. Which of the following patients is most at-risk for bed sores?

(A) An elderly patient with hypertension.

(B) An elderly patient with a history of cigarette smoking.

(C) An elderly patient with heart failure.

(D) An elderly patient with well-treated diabetes mellitus.

(101) A patient is identified as having possible mobility issues during admission. As the admitting nurse, what are the appropriate initial steps you should take to evaluate the patient?

(A) Give the patient instructions to evaluate movement.

(B) Observe the patient for signs of immobility.

(C) Read through the patient's history and examination findings.

(D) Run a quick physical examination of mobility.

(102) A patient on chronic opioid medication for cancer has become dependent on the opioid. What is the best next line of action?

(A) Reprimand the patient.

(B) Withdraw the opioid medication.

(C) Assess the patient with the CAGE questionnaire.

(D) Document the issue and inform relatives.

(103) Your patient is recommended nonpharmacological treatment for severe pain. Which of the following is not a modality of nonpharmacological treatment in the management of pain?

(A) Art.

(B) Massage.

(C) Companionship.

(D) Dietary modification.

(104) A patient with septicemia has an adverse drug reaction to the medications he is on. The patient is on the following medications: aspirin, gentamicin, and hydrochlorothiazide. Which of the following evaluations is most appropriate to identify the adverse drug reaction?

(A) Speech assessment.

(B) Hearing assessment.

(C) Visual assessment.

(D) Mobility assessment.

(105) A patient is admitted to the nephrology ward for a renal condition. Which of the following is not a primary renal/urinary tract complaint?

(A) Polyuria.

(B) Frequency.

(C) Urgency.

(D) Polydipsia.

(106) An 80-year-old presents to the ER with acute urinary retention secondary to bladder outlet obstruction due to benign enlargement of the prostate. The urinary retention is to be relieved by passing a urinary catheter. Which of the following is not ideal during the procedure?

(A) Lidocaine gel is passed into the urethra before catheterization.

(B) The self-retaining catheter inflates after passage.

(C) Phallus is adequately draped before catheterization.

(D) A smaller-sized urinary catheter is used to prevent pain and discomfort.

(107) A patient has a pelvic fracture from a traffic accident. Which of the following devices is the most appropriate for mobilization?

(A) Overhead trapeze bar.

(B) Wheelchair.

(C) Zimmer's walking frame.

(D) Axillary crutches.

(108) A patient with advanced gastric cancer had gastric bypass surgery and is experiencing dumping syndrome. Which counsel is contraindicated in this patient?

(A) Small and frequent meals.

(B) Food with high glucose content.

(C) Food rich in fiber.

(D) Moderation of fluid intake with meals.

(109) A preterm neonate admitted to the neonatal intensive unit is excessively calm and shows reduced activity. Which of the following is the least likely cause of this?

(A) Hypoglycemia.

(B) Hypothermia.

(C) Hypocalcemia.

(D) Hypoxia.

(110) A 65-year-old man was admitted for hip surgery after a hip fracture. Which of the following is not an anticipated respiratory complication of prolonged immobilization?

(A) Pulmonary fibrosis.

(B) Atelectasis.

(C) Hypostatic pneumonia.

(D) Respiratory tract infections.

(111) A 7-year-old boy is being managed for severe Guillain-Barré syndrome. Which system is not anticipated to be affected by the prolonged immobilizations associated with this condition?

(A) Integumentary.

(B) Neurological.

(C) Musculoskeletal.

(D) Gastrointestinal.

(112) Meg has acted aggressively over her last two clinic visits. She flares up whenever the nurse tells her she cannot get a higher dose of antidepressants. She claims the medicine does not work; she says she needs more medication to stay calm and gets angry when she does not take her drugs. What is the likely diagnosis?

(A) Physical dependence.

(B) Substance abuse.

(C) Drug-seeking behavior.

(D) All of the above.

(113) Which of the following is not one of the major risk factors for substance abuse?

(A) Low pain threshold.

(B) High pain threshold.

(C) Mental disorder.

(D) High risk-taking tendencies.

(114) Which of the following factors are not considered when evaluating a substance abuse client's response to a treatment plan?

(A) Achievement of sobriety.

(B) Client participation in therapy.

(C) Prevention of falls.

(D) Response to medications.

(115) A young woman lost her child a month ago and is very angry at her husband. She blames him because he failed to take her baby to the hospital in time when she was away to see a friend. She also blames her friend because they did not turn down her offer to visit despite her still nursing her baby. What coping mechanism is displayed here?

(A) Regression.

(B) Compensation.

(C) Displacement.

(D) Intellectualization.

(116) Liz wrote a suicide note, which her husband found. He called her friend, who persuaded her to visit the hospital. What is your first line of action?

(A) Use restraints on Liz.

(B) Place her on observation.

(C) Begin therapy right away.

(D) Refer Liz to a psychotherapist.

(117) When attending to your patient, you wave at a colleague and observe that your patient is very uncomfortable with your gesture. It happens twice when you wave. What do you do?

(A) Apologize for making her uncomfortable and ask what the gesture means to her.

(B) Continue as if nothing happened.

(C) Find out what the gesture means to her and apologize if need be.

(D) Stop waving when attending to the patient.

(118) What are some end-of-life concerns that patients have?

(A) Fear of the unknown.

(B) Fear of choices made.

(C) What will become of the family when they are gone.

(D) All of the above.

(119) A type of family structure where the leader makes all the decisions with little or no room for deliberation is:

(A) Democratic.

(B) Laissez-faire.

(C) Authoritarian.

(D) None of the above.

(120) Which of the following is not related to grief and loss?

(A) Worden's four tasks.

(B) Engel's stages.

(C) Sander's phases.

(D) Anna's phases.

(121) Lack of insight is an indication of:

(A) Self-efficacy.

(B) Internal locus of control.

(C) Possible non-adherence to the treatment plan.

(D) Adherence to the treatment plan.

(122) What is one important trait a nurse must exhibit when caring for patients with perception alterations?

(A) Acuity.

(B) Patience.

(C) Sound judgment.

(D) Nonjudgmental disposition.

(123) A nurse must learn to recognize nonverbal cues to manage stress effectively. Examples of these cues include:

(A) Pupil dilation.

(B) Increased respiratory rate.

(C) Sluggish movement.

(D) All of the above.

(124)Effective methods of clarification emulate which of the following?

(A) Restate, paraphrase, reflect.

(B) Challenge, probe, disagree.

(C) Focus, paraphrase, restate.

(D) Change subject, judge, stereotype.

(125) In relation to the different compatibilities of drugs, which of the following is false?

(A) Not all drugs have drug–drug interactions.

(B) Compatible drugs can be supplied in the same syringe without risk.

(C) All of the above.

(D) None of the above.

(126) You are to administer an oil- and water-based medication intramuscularly. What is the best way to approach this?

(A) Administer both separately.

(B) Mix both in the same syringe.

(C) Give one intramuscularly and the other subcutaneously.

(D) None of the above.

(127) Adverse drug reactions can be:

(A) Dose-related.

(B) Time-related.

(C) All of the above.

(D) None of the above.

(128) All of the following are blood transfusion reactions except:

(A) Fever.

(B) Chills and rigor.

(C) Tachycardia.

(D) Tachyphonia.

(129) What hematological test is most important before a patient is transfused with fresh whole blood?

(A) Full blood count and differential.

(B) Blood type and antigen screen.

(C) Blood grouping and crossmatching.

(D) Blood culture.

(130) You monitor a patient as he gets fresh whole blood. He suddenly complains of respiratory distress. Upon checking his vital signs, you notice both his heart rate and blood pressure are elevated. Your auscultatory findings are bibasal crackles. What is most likely the patient's issue?

(A) Transfusion reaction.

(B) Pulmonary embolism.

(C) Myocardial ischemia.

(D) Circulatory overload.

(131) Which of the following veins are not useful for central venous access?

(A) Subclavian.

(B) Jugular.

(C) Superior vena cava.

(D) Inferior vena cava.

(132) All of the following are complications of central venous access except:

(A) Hemothorax.

(B) Venous ulcers.

(C) Pneumothorax.

(D) Embolism.

(133) The nurse assesses the insertion site on a central line. Which finding needs to be further investigated?

(A) Biopatch and transparent dressing.

(B) A small amount of dried blood.

(C) Both A & B.

(D) Erythema and tenderness.

(134) The medication that needs the highest level of accuracy in dosing and administration is:

(A) Drug therapy in pediatrics.

(B) Intravenous fluids.

(C) Food.

(D) Vitamins.

(135) What is the equivalent volume of 500 ml in pints?

(A) 0.5 pints.

(B) 1 pint.

(C) 2 pints.

(D) 4 pints.

(136) What is the most common and convenient route of drug administration?

(A) Buccal route.

(B) Intravenous route.

(C) Transdermal route.

(D) Oral route.

(137) Which of the following should the nurse not tell a patient to then verify their medication's label?

(A) Name of the medication.

(B) Dose of the medication.

(C) Expiry date of the medication.

(D) None of the above.

(138) A patient is brought to the emergency department with third-degree burns. What is the appropriate mode of nutrition for this patient?

(A) Oral feeding.

(B) Tube feeding.

(C) Hyperalimentation.

(D) Bottle feeding.

(139) What are the main reasons for the use of total parenteral nutrition?

(A) Complete bowel rest, negative nitrogen balance, and serious medical illness or disease.

(B) Convenience.

(C) Athletic performance improvement.

(D) Routine health maintenance.

(140) What is the purpose of a hyperalimentation catheter?

(A) To deliver total parenteral nutrition.

(B) To improve athletic performance.

(C) To replace regular meals for convenience.

(D) To cure diseases.

(141) At what severity are opioids used for pain management?

(A) Mild pain.

(B) Moderate to severe pain.

(C) Chronic pain.

(D) Emotional pain.

(142) What are some common side effects of opioid medications?

(A) Drowsiness, constipation, and nausea.

(B) Increased energy and alertness.

(C) Increased appetite and weight gain.

(D) Increased blood pressure and heart rate.

(143) What is the goal of pain management?

(A) To eliminate all pain.

(B) To ignore pain.

(C) To minimize pain to a tolerable level.

(D) To maximize pain for emotional distress.

(144) Which of the following is not a potential risk of opioid medications?

(A) Addiction.

(B) Constipation.

(C) Lowered blood pressure.

(D) Respiratory depression.

(145) A patient is rushed to the emergency department. The patient is groaning in pain because he has a fractured arm. Which of the following pain management techniques is most appropriate for this patient?

(A) Use of nonopioids.

(B) Use of opioids.

(C) Cold therapy.

(D) Psychotherapy.

(146) What are some common complications of intravenous infusion therapy?

(A) Hemorrhage and emboli.

(B) Infections and phlebitis.

(C) Allergic reactions and anaphylaxis.

(D) Nausea and vomiting.

(147) Why is it important to select an appropriate vein for patients who require a blood transfusion via intravenous catheter?

(A) To minimize the risk of hematoma.

(B) To prevent fluid overload.

(C) To avoid allergic reactions.

(D) To ensure a successful blood transfusion.

(148) Why is critical thinking crucial for RNs regarding medications?

(A) Patients can be sensitive to medications.

(B) Medication administration can be complex.

(C) Medication side effects can be severe.

(D) All of the above.

(149) What are the side effects of medications?

(A) Desired therapeutic impacts.

(B) Allergic reactions.

(C) Consequences of a drug that are not expected.

(D) Severe adverse effects.

(150) Patients respond differently to medications for all of the following reasons except:

(A) Age.

(B) Health status.

(C) Eye color.

(D) Individual variability in drug metabolism.

Test 3: Answers and Explanations

(1) (B) Self-Determination Act.

The Self-Determination Act was passed by Congress in 1990. It gives patients the right to either accept or reject care upon admission to any healthcare facility. This act also gives patients the right to ask for advance directives.

(2) (B) The nurse delegating retains no responsibility for the outcome of the delegated task.

This is not true. Delegation means a task is given to another person to perform. In the nursing profession, delegation means a nurse transfers a responsibility or task to another nursing staff member but retains responsibility for the outcome of the task.

(3) (A) Skills and knowledge.

Skills and knowledge qualify a person for a job. An RN must assign jobs on this basis. Tasks must be given to staff based on the skills that they possess. There must be no sentiment about this because if a member of staff is assigned a job for which they do not possess the skills to perform, they may deliver poor quality care to the client and could make themself and the delegating nurse liable for legal action.

(4) (A) 2.

There are two types of healthcare reimbursement: prospective and retrospective.

(5) (B) ProACT model.

The Robert Wood Johnson University Hospital created this model of case management. Other models are the collaborative practice model, the case manager model, and the triad model of case management.

(6) (A) Find out what language the patient speaks and get an interpreter.

Every client has the right to accurate and easy-to-understand information about the plan for their health. Clients must know what is happening at every point in their care. If there is a communication barrier, such as a language difference, an interpreter should be provided to ensure that clients understand clearly what is being done.

(7) (C) Informed consent.

Informed consent means that patients must give full consent to whatever procedures or treatment plans are recommended, with full knowledge of the proposed treatment, including the benefits, risks, side effects, recovery, and alternatives.

(8) (A) Important decisions are made during the rounds.

Advocacy cannot happen if the nurse is absent. This is more important when critical decisions are being made, for instance, during rounds. Patients spend more time with nurses and, as such, are more comfortable discussing their concerns with them. So, the RNs can discuss a patient's concerns with doctors or other healthcare workers involved in patient management. However, this can only happen when the RN is present.

(9) (D) All of the above.

A nurse must be able to recognize the appropriate resources for common referral needs. Examples are anger management programs, social workers, self-help groups in the community for those who battle addiction or other mental health conditions, shelters and housing for clients who might be abuse victims, and elderly day care for older patients.

(10) (B) Maslow's Hierarchy of Needs.

Maslow's Hierarchy of Needs shows that the first thing to attend to is the patient's physiological needs, then their safety, security, self-esteem, and self-actualization.

(11) (A) Highest risk areas.

The best areas for quality improvement are those with the highest risk, monetary and human resource costs, and volume, which are the most vulnerable to problems. Performance improvement aims to enhance and improve the quality and outcomes of care. This increases the efficiency of patient care and reduces costs, risks, and liabilities.

(12) (B) Specific variance.

A specific variance occurs whenever the faulty process is carried out. It is predictable and usually occurs when a specific part of the process is faulty or vulnerable to human error.

(13) (C) Method de jour.

Performance improvement activities can be done through many methods, some of which include the PDCA cycle, which involves Planning, Doing, Checking, and

Acting; the Six Sigma method, which involves problem definition measurement, analysis of data, improvements to make and control; and the method de jour.

(14) (C) Nursing assistants.

LPNs are licensed healthcare professionals. They provide a wide variety of nursing care services in many different healthcare settings. RNs are licensed healthcare personnel who are trained to deliver nursing care in several healthcare settings. Nursing assistants/patient care technicians are non-licensed assistants who help nurses to provide direct and indirect care.

(15) (C) Physical therapist.

Physical therapists are licensed healthcare personnel that provide medical interventions concerned with a patient's functional abilities. They consider factors like strength, gait, and mobility and use tools like walkers and exercise routines to achieve their outcomes.

(16) (C) Approach-Avoidance.

Here, the choices that can resolve the conflict are not completely satisfactory to both parties, but neither are they completely unsatisfactory.

(17) (D) All of the above.

Some of the most common causes of conflict in healthcare settings are disrespect, overworking, unfair distribution of roles or duties, ill health, patient loss, negligence, limited resources, poor remuneration, poor communication skills, and different personality types.

(18) (C) I, III, II.

Doctors on call should be informed. Anti-tetanus serum/tetanus toxoid should be given, and materials for suturing should be prepared. The patient also requires an X-ray.

(19) (A) Pathophysiology.

The pathophysiology of the disease should guide the delivery of care. The presentation is important but does not always determine how care is administered. Some presentations might be dramatic but not urgent. Some patients also exaggerate their symptoms. Hence, knowledge of disease conditions should guide how care is delivered, not subjective displays or responses.

(20) (C) A and B.

Scenarios like this should be documented, including the counseling and the refusal, and reported to appropriate authorities for follow-up. A nurse should not forcefully immunize a child against the wishes of the parents and caregiver. The parent is the major consent giver for minors.

(21) (D) All of the above.

The fundamental responsibility of the nurse is to prevent illness, promote health, restore health, and alleviate suffering.

(22) (D) 09/10/20 1145 hrs. IV acetaminophen 300 mg STAT given. Patient reports pain as 2/10.

The right way to input information for clients is the date, time, drug and correct route of administration, dose, frequency, and assessment of the patient.

(23) (B) "I am sorry. I cannot give out such information about my clients."

Let your friend know that you cannot give out such information. It is against HIPAA to give out information to a person whose input is not necessary to the care of the patient, either directly or indirectly. Suggest your friend call and ask her brother or his wife.

(24) (B) Speak Spanish and reassure the patient that you will get an interpreter with a better command of the language.

You should speak whatever Spanish is possible and allow the patient to calm down. Then you can go get an interpreter with a better command of the language. If you go ahead and try to interpret, there might be a misunderstanding or a loss of the message to be passed across.

(25) (B) Document and report it.

Abuse of clients, gunshot wounds, road traffic accidents, burns, harmful diseases, or cases of food poisoning should be reported. VOs can only be used during emergencies. Since this is not an emergency, the physician can request another physician who is around to document the order so it can be given.

(26) (B) IV morphine 150 mg STAT for postoperative pain.

Most likely this is an incorrect dosage. IV morphine is usually given between 4 mg to 10 mg over three or four times daily or PRN. The dose of 150 mg STAT is not correct.

(27) (C) Prepare for craniotomy.

Informed consent is not needed when a delay would cause harm or death to the patient. In this case, a search for the patient's relatives can result in a waste of precious time. This patient needs to receive care as soon as possible. The law allows this kind of scenario without informed consent.

(28) (C) Hormonal profile.

A hormonal profile test is a blood test that is used to detect hormonal imbalances and fertility issues in women. It assesses the quantity of estrogen, progesterone, thyroid hormones, follicle-stimulating hormone, and testosterone. For this case, a doctor might also include prolactin as one of the hormones to test for.

(29) (C) All risks are modifiable.

Biologically, some risks are evident based on race, age, and sex and cannot be modified. For instance, the female sex has a higher chance of breast cancer than the male sex.

(30) (D) None of the above.

There are several health risks that individuals are exposed to daily. Some of these risks are based on the patients' age, socioeconomic status, hobbies, lifestyle choices, location, and population. It is the nurse's responsibility to assess clients for possible health risks that they are exposed to knowingly or unknowingly.

(31) (C) Physical readiness.

Physical readiness involves the measures of ability, the complexity of the task, the effect of the environment, the health status of the individual, and sex. The measures of physical ability determine whether a patient is ready to learn or not. A patient with a motor impairment might find it difficult to perform some fine movements and might not be ready to learn things such as how to clean a surgical wound appropriately.

(32) (D) A and C.

From time to time, nurses have to provide education to help achieve these objectives of developing health characteristics. When these needs are identified, the nurse can devise a plan to intervene as needed. Intervention might involve educating community members via oral presentations, counseling, and guidance for individuals or even multidisciplinary cooperation. Policy approval is not the duty of a nurse.

(33) (B) It is graded from 0 to 5.

The New Ballard scale is based on both physical maturity and the maturity of the neuromuscular system. It is graded from -1 to 5 and measures the following parameters: posture, square window (the movement of the wrist), arm recoil, scarf sign, and heel-to-ear movement.

(34) (A) Erikson's initiative vs. guilt stage.

Erikson's initiative vs. guilt stage coincides with the preschooler age (three to five years). At this stage, children refine their motor skills. This is the stage at which disabilities that affect development are more obvious.

(35) (A) Young adults.

Young adults between 19 and 35 are at the intimacy vs. isolation stage, according to Erikson. Here, they begin to form closer, stronger relationships with other people.

This stage is also characterized by a search for purpose in life and the development of healthy coping mechanisms to deal with the demands of work, relationships, and other commitments.

(36) (D) B and C.

Musculoskeletal changes in the elderly include a decrease in muscle mass, muscle tone and strength, degenerating joints and bones, and reductions in intervertebral disc spaces.

(37) (C) December 25, 2023.

The EDD is calculated as 40 weeks after the last menstrual period (LMP). It can be used in clinical settings to estimate the EDD. However, the most reliable method to estimate the EDD is the early ultrasound taken in the first trimester of pregnancy.

(38) (D) All of the above.

The OFC of the newborn should increase at an average rate of 2 cm per month for the first three months, then 1 cm per month for the next six months. The length should also increase at a rate of about 2.5 cm per month for the first six months and about 1.3 cm for the last six months of the first year. If a child is not feeding well, it should be checked as soon as possible.

(39) (D) Several times a day.

The umbilical cord stump usually falls off a newborn within one to two weeks after birth. Until it falls off, the area should be kept clean and dry and be cleaned several times a day. This helps prevent infection. After each diaper change, the area around the cord should be cleaned with a cotton swab dipped in warm water, then dried thoroughly.

(40) (A) Educate her.

The only way to ascertain for sure that a woman is breastfeeding her child right is to watch her do it, especially if this is her first child. This type of learning ensures that the mother uses the right technique that will not harm her or the baby over time.

(41) (A) The physical and social setting in which nursing care is provided.

The client care environment refers to the physical and social setting in which nursing care is provided. To assess the client care environment, consider factors such as safety, comfort, privacy, and cultural sensitivity.

(42) (B) Assess the quality of the client's home environment.

The healthcare environment must be regulated to minimize falls and other injuries to ensure a safe client care environment. Materials and equipment used should be sterile or properly disinfected before reuse, and all allergens must be removed. The environment should also be checked for factors that can trigger self-harm or aggression in patients. It is not a nurse's responsibility to examine the client's home environment.

(43) (A) Bedside monitors.

Bedside monitors are the most effective for monitoring clients who are unconscious and unable to use other methods to signal staff members.

(44) (C) The Sims position is not the same as the semi-prone position.

This is false. The Sims position is also known as the semi-prone position and is halfway between the prone and lateral positions.

(45) (B) 2.

Having at least two distinct identifiers for each client besides their room number is recommended.

(46) (D) None of the above.

Internal disasters are those that occur within the confines of medical facilities, such as fire hazards, workplace violence, radiation contamination, building collapse, and other utility failures.

(47) (A) The most critical situations be attended to first.

During triage, the nurse should assess patients' situations from most critical to least critical. Critical situations should be attended to first, and in situations of equipment and bed space shortage, noncritical patients may be treated and discharged immediately.

(48) (D) All of the above.

Ergonomic principles can be applied when providing healthcare. These will help offer comfort to clients and help them maintain the right posture, balance, body alignment, and body movement as they use assistive devices and other facilities like beds and stretchers. Nurses should keep in mind ergonomic principles and body mechanics when providing care to clients and helping them use assistive devices.

(49) (B) Provide a secure base for better balance.

Keep your feet apart to provide a secure base to support yourself when lifting.

(50) (B) A client who mostly maintains the same position due to immobility or weakness in certain muscle groups.

Clients who maintain the same position over time have a high risk of repetitive stress injury due to the overuse of certain muscles or muscle groups.

(51) (D) To ensure clients have an appropriate home environment for quick response and adjustment to new health challenges.

Nurses must strongly consider client pathophysiology and the uniqueness of each client's situation when they offer solutions to ensure clients have an appropriate home environment for quick response and adjustment to new health challenges.

(52) (B) Used hospital beddings.

Biohazardous material includes items that have been contaminated with biological waste that can become harmful to humans. Used hospital bedding, tubes containing bodily fluids and excretions, and used needles are all examples of biohazardous waste.

(53) (C) All of the above.

Details that should be included in formal reports include the date, time, and place where the event happened, brief background information on what triggered the event, the name of people affected by the event, and the nature of the injuries sustained.

(54) (C) Practitioner, system, and patient.

The events that should be reported include practitioner variance, system or institutional variance, and patient variance.

(55) (C) Preventive and infection control measures utilized to combat and inhibit the spread of specific infections.

Transmission-based precautions are additional infection prevention measures used for patients who have known or suspected infectious diseases. Precautions are based on the disease's mode of transmission.

(56) (D) All of the above.

RNs directly and indirectly educate clients and staff members on infection prevention and control measures. They assess the educational needs of these groups and plan educational activities to meet those needs. They also evaluate the impact and effectiveness of such educational sessions on infection prevention and control.

(57) (B) Provide special care only when there is an infection outbreak.

Immunocompromised clients should be isolated from other people until they have attained some level of recovery and immunity, and stringent infection control measures should be practiced. This includes protecting them from infections that might not pose a threat to non-compromised clients.

(58) (C) Move away from the sterile field before they cough or sneeze.

Coughing or sneezing over the sterile field contaminates it, so the nurse should move away from the sterile field before they cough or sneeze. The nurse should never have the sterile field below the waist level. The nurse should lean over or turn their back to the sterile field.

(59) (C) To prevent safety threats such as falls.

Restraints and safety devices may be required when mobility can increase the risk of falls, suicide attempts, or harm to others.

(60) (D) Isolation in one room with no means of exit.

Different kinds of restraints are appropriate in different situations. These include belts, jackets, and other devices that prevent limb movement, physical restraint of a patient to restrict movement, and medicine that keeps the patient immobile. However, isolating the patient in one room with no means of exit is not an appropriate type of restraint.

(61) (C) Lateral aspect of the wrist.

Knowledge of the anatomy of the body and the pathophysiology of diseases is critical for those who must notice and respond to abnormal vital signs. For instance, knowledge of anatomy helps a nurse read the radial pulse on the lateral side of the wrist. The radial pulse gives the pulse rate of the individual. The average in an adult is 70 bpm.

(62) (B) 2/3 of the upper arm.

While there are varying schools of thought, most textbooks and experienced practitioners recommend the blood pressure cuff should cover two-thirds of the upper arm's length. This upper arm length is defined as the distance between the axilla and the antecubital fossa. The wrong cuff size can affect the result of the blood pressure measurement.

(63) (C) Strip and meter.

The nurse should use the right strip and meter to do blood glucose testing.

(64) (D) Head.

ECG leads are placed on the upper limbs, chest, and lower limbs.

(65) (B) To compare with patient values.

Standardized values are essential in laboratory investigations. They form a baseline with which we can compare patient values to determine quantities that are depressed, normal, or elevated. They also help to monitor values and determine whether the treatment plan is beneficial to the patient or not.

(66) (D) All of the above.

A tourniquet is used in venipuncture to briefly arrest blood flow back to the heart, which makes the veins engorged and more visible so that the cannula can be easily inserted. The tourniquet is also used to ensure the skin is taut around the region for the venipuncture.

(67) (D) Respiratory tract infections.

Urine is routinely collected for urinary tract infections, sexually transmitted infections, and renal diseases. Urine is not routinely collected for investigations of respiratory tract infections.

(68) (D) A and B.

After nurses identify these patients, nurses are responsible for educating them on how to avoid complications of their diseases and how to avoid developing others they are at risk of. This education includes lifestyle choices and their impact, which can be immediate, temporary, longer, or permanent.

(69) (B) Choice of diet.

Patients with a family history or relatives with skin cancer are also at risk. Patients whose occupation exposes them to ultraviolet radiation are also predisposed to skin cancers. Patients with a personal history of skin cancer are at risk. No significant study links diet as a major risk factor for skin cancer.

(70) (A) Hypotension.

Hypotension is when blood pressure falls below normal values, usually less than 90/60 mmHg. Hypertension with a corresponding pulse might later happen when the body is trying to adapt. Patients might also experience confusion, weakness, blurred vision, or fainting.

(71) (C) High Fowler's position.

In this position, the patient is seated upright with the upper body positioned between 60 and 90 degrees. This position greatly reduces the risk of regurgitation and aspiration.

(72) (D) 15–30 degrees.

At 15–30 degrees, the cannula can be easily advanced into the vein. This angle also allows for easy visualization of the flashback of blood once the cannula is in the vein.

(73) (C) Note the volume of the urine.

Removal of the catheter must be done with aseptic techniques. Most importantly, the catheter should be removed gently, disconnected from the urine bag, and properly disposed of. The contents must be measured before the bag is emptied.

(74) (C) 0–5.

The nurse can assess the muscles and score them from 0–5. The muscles score zero if there's no visible contraction and score five (full power) if there's a full contraction against high resistance levels. A zero score can be due to either neurological or musculoskeletal anomalies.

(75) (C) 12.

The 12 cranial nerves include the olfactory nerve (CN I); the optic nerve (CN II); the oculomotor nerve (CN III); the trochlear nerve (CN IV); the trigeminal nerve (CN V); the abducens nerve (CN VI); the facial nerve (CN VII); the vestibulocochlear nerve (CN VIII); the glossopharyngeal nerve (CN IX); the vagus nerve (CN X); the spinal accessory nerve (CN XI); and the hypoglossal nerve (CN XII).

(76) (A) They're always medical.

Therapeutic procedures are not always medical. The modality of the therapeutic procedure employed depends on the condition. But surgical procedures are sometimes the only form of therapy that can address a condition, such as tumors.

(77) (A) To help educate the patient.

How to educate the patient about the treatment procedure is a skill every nurse should have. A nurse should explain each procedure's benefits, risks, and side effects. Every patient also has the right to forfeit or reject a treatment. Lastly, a nurse must get informed consent before they begin a treatment.

(78) (A) Hepatitis B.

Hepatitis B is the only illness in this question transmitted by needle pricks. Hepatitis A is transmitted by the fecal-oral route. Leukemia is a disease of the white blood cells, which can be due to several etiologies, but not needle pricks. Other diseases that can be transmitted by needle pricks include HIV/AIDS and Hepatitis C.

(79) (A) Thoughts, behaviors, and emotions.

Coping mechanisms are thoughts, behaviors, and emotions that patients use to adapt to and cope with stress. Some of these mechanisms can be healthy, while others are maladaptive.

(80) (D) Check blood levels in the lab.

All other ways are subjective and can be affected by lighting conditions, the nurse's experience, and the patient's skin color. But the blood levels of bilirubin shown by lab tests can accurately tell whether the bilirubin levels are elevated. In the clinical setting, other methods, such as the skin color and color of the eyes, can be used to detect hyperbilirubinemia, but they must be confirmed by a bilirubin test.

(81) (A) Fine needle aspiration and core needle biopsy.

Fine needle aspiration (FNA) is a minimally invasive diagnostic procedure that involves the insertion of a fine hollow needle into a mass or lump to obtain samples, which are then stained and observed. Core needle biopsy is an invasive diagnostic procedure that uses a slightly larger needle to obtain more tissue from masses. It is generally preferred to the FNA.

(82) (C) Handwashing.

Bacteria and microbes can hide in the inner lining of ventilator tubes and cause infections in patients. Pneumonia is a common disease acquired by patients on ventilators. Basic aseptic techniques like handwashing can prevent the transfer of bacteria to patients.

(83) (B) Suctioning cannot be done more than once.

This is false. Suctioning is the mechanical aspiration of pulmonary secretions from the airways. Oxygen is administered before suctioning to maintain the airways during suctioning. A sterile glove is worn, and the tip of the suction catheter is lubricated. The catheter is slowly advanced into the patient's airways to remove secretions. This process can be repeated until the airways are clear.

(84) (D) Hematomas.

A hematoma refers to a collection of blood, mostly clotted in a closed cavity or space. Hematomas usually result from the rupture of an artery or vein within a tissue, an organ, or a cavity. Hematomas can form a lump under the skin that can be felt, but they are not open wounds. Abrasions, punctures, and gunshot wounds are all open wounds.

(85) (D) A and B.

The patient is monitored after surgery by the nurse. The vital signs are first examined. The pulse rate and blood pressure are measured. The respiratory system is also examined. Patients in recovery from general anesthesia are at risk of dysphagia and laryngospasms. They might also feel some lightheadedness and drowsiness, which will eventually wear off. So patients should be reassured.

(86) (D) Acute rhinitis.

Postural drainage is very useful in patients with conditions that produce excessive secretions, such as COPD or bronchiectasis. Acute rhinitis does not produce copious secretions and is not an indication of postural drainage.

(87) (C) Hemodialysis and peritoneal dialysis.

Dialysis replaces the function of the kidney. There are two types of dialysis: hemodialysis and peritoneal dialysis. Hemodialysis is a form of dialysis via an AV fistula or a central vascular line. An AV is a connection between an artery and vein and is done three months before the dialysis to allow for maturity. Peritoneal dialysis is done by passing a catheter into the peritoneal space. This option is for patients who are at risk of complications from medications given on hemodialysis.

(88) (A) The kidneys' ultrafiltration function.

As a result of failure, the kidneys cannot filter waste products for excretion. Therefore, waste products accumulate in the body, which is dangerous to the patient. Dialysis helps to remove these waste products. It replaces the ultrafiltration function of the kidneys to clear waste products from the body and balance the pH of the blood.

(89) (D) Stage V.

There are five stages of renal failure or chronic kidney disease. Stage I presents with a normal GFR of 90 ml/min or higher. Stage II is mild CKD with GR of 60–89 ml/min. Stage III is moderate CKD with GFR of 30–59 ml/min. Stage 4 is Severe CKD with GFR of 15–29 ml/min. Stage 5 is the end stage CKD with GFR of < 15 ml/min. End-stage CKD is where dialysis or renal transplant is needed.

(90) (B) Na.

Sodium (Na) is the most abundant extracellular cation, and it is heavily involved in muscular contraction. Potassium (K) is the most abundant intracellular cation. Magnesium is a dominant intracellular ion that also regulates several signaling pathways and channels. It is also involved in preventing continuous muscular contractions. Chlorine is an anion.

(91) (D) None of the above.

Sodium and potassium are the major cations involved in muscular contraction, while calcium is involved in both cardiac and muscular contraction.

(92) (A) Stop the fluid infusion.

The patient is most likely suffering from fluid overload due to the infusion that is being received. Therefore, the first step is to stop the infusion. The next step would be to commence the patient on Lasix.

(93) (B) Resuscitation.

Fluid resuscitation is the first line of treatment in hypovolemia. Infusion of intravenous fluids like ringer's lactate can expand the blood volume.

(94) (D) Common interosseous artery.

Arterial lines can be placed in various arteries like the femoral, brachial and radial arteries. These lines are inserted via a surgical procedure to monitor the patient's blood pressure. Arterial lines can also be used to obtain frequent blood samples.

(95) (D) All of the above.

The nurse should be aware of the potential complications of having a pacemaker. Complications include pneumothorax, hemothorax, perforation of the pacemaker lead and cardiac tamponade.

(96) (B) Interpretation of ECG.

When there is a problem with the patient's ECG, the nurse has to interpret the ECG and decide on the next course of action.

(97) (D) All of the above.

The nurse should be able to explain how the disease process began. Patients should be told about the risk factors predisposing them to the disease. Nurses should inform patients about factors that can be changed and reduce the chances of developing the illness. The signs and symptoms of the disease should be explained to the patients so they can report to the doctor if they see any.

(98) (D) B and C.

Illness management begins with educating the patient about acute and chronic conditions. The education of patients includes information about the pathophysiology of the disease condition.

(99) (D) Arrhythmias.

Arrhythmias are mostly seen in hyperkalemia. Hypernatremia is an elevation of the sodium level above the usual standard. Hypernatremia can arise from several illnesses and conditions like diabetes insipidus, diarrhea, vomiting and Cushing's syndrome. Features of hypernatremia include thirst, agitation, restlessness and confusion.

(100) (C) An elderly patient with heart failure.

An elderly patient with heart failure has the highest risk of developing bed sores because of reduced tissue perfusion and reduced mobility.

(101) (B) Observation of the patient for signs of immobility.

The first step in the evaluation of the patient for immobility begins with observation. Observation can reveal mobility issues that the patient might not be aware of.

(102) (C) Assess the patient using the CAGE questionnaire.

The best line of action is to assess the patient using the CAGE questionnaire to assess dependency.

(103) (D) Dietary modification.

Dietary modification is not a modality in the nonpharmacological management of pain. Nonpharmacological modalities include arts, music, companionship, massage, counseling, exercise and drama.

(104) (B) Hearing assessment.

Aspirin, gentamicin and hydrochlorothiazide are known to have adverse effects of ototoxicity. Hence a hearing assessment is the most appropriate evaluation in this case.

(105) (D) Polydipsia.

Polydipsia is not a primary urinary complaint.

(106) (C) Phallus is adequately draped before catheterization.

For acute urinary retention, the primary focus is on ensuring the procedure is carried out effectively and safely, with minimal discomfort for the patient. Although maintaining dignity and privacy is important, the use of the term "adequately draped" in this context is less relevant and not ideal as a priority during the procedure.

(107) (A) Overhead trapeze bar.

An overhead trapeze bar is the best device as the patient's pelvic mobilization is limited to prevent further injury.

(108) (B) Food with high glucose content.

Intake of high glucose meals will exacerbate dumping syndrome.

(109) (C) Hypocalcemia.

Hypocalcemia is unlikely to induce this state in the preterm neonate compared to the other above diagnoses. It should, however, be noted that hypocalcemia is a common problem of preterm neonates.

(110) (A) Pulmonary fibrosis.

Pulmonary fibrosis is not an anticipated respiratory complication of prolonged immobilization. Respiratory complications of prolonged immobilization include respiratory infections, atelectasis, hypostatic pneumonia, shallow respiration and decreased respiratory movement.

(111) (B) Neurological.

The neurological system is unlikely to be affected by prolonged immobilization. Systems commonly affected in prolonged immobilization include the integumentary system, pressure sores; musculoskeletal system, muscle atrophy; gastrointestinal system, constipation; and urinary system, urine stasis and infection.

(112) (D) All of the above.

She wants more drugs, which is drug-seeking behavior and is exhibiting withdrawal symptoms when she does not take her drugs, pointing to physical dependence.

(113) (B) High pain threshold.

Risk factors for substance abuse include a low pain threshold, several failed attempts at suicide, a high tendency to take risks, a high tendency to self-medicate and a concurrent mental disorder.

(114) (C) Prevention of falls.

Some things to be considered include achieving sobriety, participation in therapy and response to medications. Prevention of falls is not a factor that is considered when evaluating a treatment plan.

(115) (C) Displacement.

Displacement is a coping mechanism in which a client transfers anger, aggression or feelings of frustration at one person onto another person or object. In the question, the woman has transferred her anger and frustration at her baby's death onto her husband and friend as a way of coping with the fact that her baby died while she was not around.

(116) (B) Place her on observation.

Any threats of suicide or violence should not be handled lightly. The patient should be constantly observed, and restraints can be used if necessary.

(117) (A) Apologize for making her uncomfortable and ask what the gesture means to her.

A nurse must respect all cultures as long as it does not harm the client or other clients.

(118) (D) All of the above.

Patients might have psychological needs which can be diverse. They might battle with confusion, sleep disturbances and depression.

(119) (C) Authoritarian.

Some families operate in an authoritarian structure where the leader makes all the decisions with little or no room for deliberation among family members. Others run a democratic structure where all family members can deliberate on decisions to be made. Some other families run a laissez-faire leadership where individuals within the family unit are left to make their own decisions while the leaders support and provide the needed resources.

(120) (D) Anna's phases.

Grief models include Sander's phases of bereavement, which involve shock, awareness of loss, conservation, withdrawal, healing or turning point and renewal. Worden's four tasks of mourning include accepting the loss, coping with the loss, altering the environment to cope with the loss and resuming a healthy life. Engel's stages of grieving involve shock and disbelief, developing awareness, restitution, resolution of the loss, idealization and outcome.

(121) (C) Possible non-adherence to the treatment plan.

Some of the parameters to look out for in evaluating a client's adherence include the participation of the client in the plan or not, previous experiences where a similar treatment plan did not work, lack of insight of the client, denial, self-efficacy, internal locus of control and side effects of the plan.

(122) (D) Nonjudgmental disposition.

Nursing care for patients with alterations or perception loss must be done in a nonjudgmental manner, no matter what the clients say or the behaviors they display.

(123) (D) All of the above.

For nurses to effectively manage stress, they must be able to recognize nonverbal cues and respond appropriately. Using Hans Selye's general adaptation theory, some of the cues from the alarm stage are pupil dilation, increased heart rate, respiratory rate, glucose consumption, cardiac output and increased adrenaline and cortisol levels with attendant manifestations. The resistance stage is marked by increased cardiac output and a maintained respiratory rate and blood pressure increase. The third stage is exhaustion. Other signs to look out for include loss of consciousness, hyperglycemia and hypoglycemia.

(124) (A) Restating, paraphrasing, reflecting.

Restating involves repeating exactly what the client said to clarify what was said. Reflecting involves a reflection of what the client is conveying beyond the words that are said. Paraphrasing involves a nurse saying what they understood from what the client said in their own words.

(125) (D) None of the above.

Compatible drugs can be mixed in the same syringe, and not all drugs have drug-drug interactions.

(126) (A) Administer both separately.

Oil and water don't mix, so a colloid is formed, so this makes B wrong. Option C was not part of the question as the question was specifically intramuscular.

(127) (C) All of the above.

Adverse drug reactions are classified into six types: dose-related (augmented), non-dose-related (bizarre), dose-related and time-related (chronic), time-related (delayed), withdrawal (end of use) and failure of therapy (failure).

(128) (D) Tachyphonia.

Tachyphonia is not a blood transfusion reaction. A blood transfusion reaction is characterized by fever, nausea, anxiety, chills, warm, flushed skin and other symptoms.

(129) (C) Blood grouping and crossmatching.

Blood grouping and crossmatching should be done to ensure compatibility between the whole blood donor and recipient.

(130) (D) Circulatory overload.

Hypertension, respiratory distress, tachycardia and bibasal crackles (pulmonary edema) are all signs and symptoms of circulatory overload. Patients with pulmonary embolism often have sudden onset shortness of breath, chest pain and sinus tachycardia as the most common ECG findings. Patients with transfusion reactions often present with itching, chills, urticaria and fever.

(131) (D) Inferior vena cava.

Central venous catheters are placed into the heart's right atrium via the superior vena cava. Central venous catheters can be introduced into the superior vena cava via a peripheral vein, as with a PICC, or via the subclavian or jugular vein. The inferior vena cava is not involved.

(132) (B) Venous ulcers.

Venous ulcers are complications commonly seen on IV catheters placed in the lower extremities. Central venous catheter insertion can cause complications such as infection, pneumothorax, hemothorax, thrombosis and embolism.

(133) (D) Erythema and tenderness.

This signifies an inflammatory response that may be due to an infection.

(134) (A) Drug therapy in pediatrics.

Pediatric patients require especially accurate dosing due to their smaller size and the way their bodies metabolize medications. Small deviations from the appropriate dose can result in either therapeutic failure or toxicity. Therefore, you should adjust doses based on the child’s weight and sometimes the child’s body surface area.

(135) (B) 1 pint.

One pint is equal to 16 ounces of fluid, and 1 ounce is equal to 30 ml. Therefore, 1 pint is equal to 16 x 30 = 480 ml. So, 500 ml is slightly more than 1 pint.

(136) (D) Oral route.

The oral route of drug administration is the most common, most accessible and most convenient for patients. It is usually the first choice, except when a patient cannot tolerate it or when swift action is needed, then the intravenous route can be considered.

(137) (D) None of the above.

The name of the medication, dose and expiration date should all be verified.

(138) (C) Hyperalimentation.

Total parenteral nutrition is most often used for patients who require complete bowel rest.

(139) (A) Complete bowel rest, negative nitrogen balance, serious medical illness or disease.

The main reasons for using total parenteral nutrition are complete bowel rest, negative nitrogen balance and serious medical illness or disease.

(140) (A) To deliver total parenteral nutrition.

The purpose of a hyperalimentation catheter is to deliver total parenteral nutrition.

(141) (B) Moderate to severe pain.

Opioids are used to treat moderate to severe pain.

(142) (A) Drowsiness, constipation and nausea.

The common side effects of opioid medications include drowsiness, constipation and nausea.

(143) (C) To minimize pain to a tolerable level.

The goal of pain management is to minimize pain to a tolerable level.

(144) (C) Lowered blood pressure.

Some of the potential risks of opioid medications include addiction, constipation and respiratory depression. Reduction in blood pressure is, however, not one of the risks of opioid use.

(145) (B) Use of opioids.

Opioids are used to manage moderate to severe pain.

(146) (B) Infections and phlebitis.

Common complications from intravenous infusion therapy include infections, phlebitis, fluid overload and hematoma.

(147) (D) To ensure successful blood transfusion.

Selecting an appropriate vein is important to ensure a successful blood transfusion. If a vein is not patent enough, the blood transfusion can be affected. If the vein is also not good enough, it can lead to the formation of a hematoma.

(148) (D) All of the above.

The ability to think critically is important for RNs because some patients are given pharmaceuticals for a short time for acute sickness. In contrast, others may take medications for a chronic health issue for an extended time. Prescription pharmaceuticals, over-the-counter medications, vitamins, supplements and alternative medications are examples of these medications.

(149) (C) Consequences of a drug that are not expected.

The term “side effects” refers to all the consequences of a drug that are not the expected therapeutic impact of the medication. They are also known as adverse reactions or adverse effects.

(150) (C) Eye color.

Patients may respond differently due to factors such as age, health status, genetics and individual variability in drug metabolism. Eye color will not affect drug metabolism.

Test 4: Questions

1. One of the patients in your ward complained of severe headaches. You checked her blood pressure and it was 170/150 mmhg. She said she had used the BP medications which had been given to her the previous week. You check her charts and observe that her blood pressure has been uncontrolled since she changed her medications last week. What do you do?

(A) Inform physicians.

(B) Confirm that the patient has been taking medications correctly.

(C) Ask the patient to continue medications.

(D) A and B.

2. Mrs. Parker is currently unconscious and has to undergo a craniotomy for a suspected hematoma. This procedure was not included in her living will. What should be done?

(A) Contact her husband to decide.

(B) Let her healthcare proxy decide.

(C) Contact her next of kin.

(D) All of the above.

3. Which of the following is not included in the Self-Determination Act?

(A) Right to accept care on admission.

(B) Right to reject care on admission.

(C) Right to reject advance directives.

(D) Right to ask for advance directives.

4. Which of the following is not involved in advocacy?

(A) Advocating for staff members.

(B) Listening to patients.

(C) Observing nonverbal cues.

(D) None of the above.

5. Which of the following should not be mentioned in discussing specified treatment modalities?

(A) The benefits of a procedure.

(B) The side effects of a procedure.

(C) The personnel carrying out the procedure.

(D) None of the above.

6. How many rights of delegation have been proposed by the American Nurses Association?

(A) 4.

(B) 5.

(C) 6.

(D) 7.

7. For the right circumstances, what is the major question to ask?

(A) Is the circumstance right for delegation in this patient?

(B) What is the state of the patient?

(C) Who would be held accountable for the outcome of this task?

(D) What is the state of the health care personnel?

8. A 65-year-old patient is currently on oxygen at 10 l/min. $SPO2 = 70\%$, PR = 120 bpm, and BP = 90/60 mmhg. Which of the following is correct?

(A) All tasks for this patient should be delegated.

(B) Some tasks for this patient can be delegated.

(C) No tasks for this patient can be delegated.

(D) None of the above.

9. Which of the following frameworks is in the right order?

(A) Airway, breathing, circulatory.

(B) Self-esteem, safety, physiological needs, security, self-actualization.

(C) Breathing airway, circulatory.

(D) Circulatory, airway, breathing.

10. Abe is to be transferred to another hospital for more expert management. What is the role of the nurse here?

(A) The nurse has no active role.

(B) Ensure the client and family are educated on the plan of care.

(C) Update the patient's plan of care.

(D) B and C.

11. The social security number of a patient is protected by:

(A) HIPAA.

(B) The Patient's Bill of Rights.

(C) The Self-Determination Act.

(D) All of the above.

12. Patients have the right to know all available treatment options and decide which they want to choose. They also have a right to select who can choose treatments for them when they are not able to make such decisions. This is known as the right to:

(A) Confidentiality.

(B) Informed consent.

(C) Informed decisions.

(D) Client responsibilities.

13. A 78-year-old woman has been admitted for stroke management and her condition has become more unstable. What are the things a nurse must observe?

(A) Vital signs.

(B) Adverse drug events.

(C) Mood changes.

(D) All of the above.

14. Specimen collection can be performed by:

(A) Licensed practical nurses.

(B) Patient care technicians.

(C) Nursing supervisors.

(D) A and B.

15. What group of healthcare workers are primarily involved in appropriately moving the patient along the continuum of care?

(A) Occupational therapists.

(B) Physical therapists.

(C) Cardiologists.

(D) Social workers.

16. Which is not part of the nursing process?

(A) Planning.

(B) Assessing.

(C) Implanting.

(D) None of the above.

17. Two of the nursing staff under you have a disagreement over their work hours. The nurse who feels cheated stops speaking to the other staff member, while the other party is ignoring the issue. Which of the following methods can be used to resolve the conflict?

(A) Talk to other nurses about the problem.

(B) Avoid the issue when they are around.

(C) Promote competition.

(D) Suggest a compromise.

18. What is the role of the director of nursing in patient care?

(A) Indirect.

(B) Direct.

(C) Mixed.

(D) None of the above.

19. One of your staff has not logged out of the computer even though she has finished what she is doing. What is this an example of?

(A) She has violated patient rights according to HIPAA.

(B) She has violated patient rights according to the Patient's Bill of Rights.

(C) She has violated the anatomical act.

(D) All of the above.

20. What are the 5P's in the continuity of care?

(A) Patient, Purpose, Problems, Perspective, Privileges.

(B) Precision, Purpose, Patient, Problems, Perspective.

(C) Patient, Plan, Purpose, Problems, Precautions.

(D) None of the above.

21. Which of the following is not involved in the management of care?

(A) Provision of nursing care.

(B) Coordination of nursing care.

(C) Safe health care delivery setting.

(D) None of the above.

22. What is the fundamental responsibility of a nurse?

(A) Prevent illness.

(B) Promote peace.

(C) Settle conflicts.

(D) All of the above.

23. In end-of-life scenarios, what roles do nurses play?

(A) Meet patients' physical needs.

(B) Educate patients and relatives.

(C) Provide psychological help.

(D) All of the above.

24. What is the first thing to do when you receive a patient order?

(A) Verification.

(B) Planning.

(C) Evaluation.

(D) Implementation.

25. What principle requires that the nurse always act in the best interest of the patient?

(A) Beneficence.

(B) Maleficence.

(C) Confidentiality.

(D) Information.

26. Which of the following is involved in the elimination of falls?

(A) Safety management.

(B) Risk management.

(C) Outcome measures.

(D) All of the above.

27. What comprises the Six Sigma Method?

(A) Patient, prevention, planning, perspective purpose, proactiveness.

(B) Problem definition, measurement, data analysis, improvements, and control.

(C) Verbal communication, names, departments, written documents, forms, and reports.

(D) None of the above.

28. A 35-year-old patient who is being referred on account of schizophrenia might need which of the following services?

(A) Shelters.

(B) Daycare.

(C) Social workers.

(D) Self-help groups.

29. Which of the following is not typically caused by an allergy?

(A) Tachycardia.

(B) Bradycardia.

(C) Chest tightness.

(D) None of the above.

30. An 80-year-old woman is admitted into the ward. What is not a major risk factor for falls or accidents?

(A) Developmental stage.

(B) Elderly.

(C) Mental status.

(D) Hunger.

31. Which method of staff signaling is most effective in the ICU?

(A) Call bell.

(B) Intercom.

(C) Bedside monitors.

(D) All of the above.

32. A nurse in your ward gave medication to the wrong patient. How can this be stopped from happening again?

(A) Have more than two distinct identifiers.

(B) Verify the accuracy of a treatment order.

(C) A and B.

(D) None of the above.

33. A patient presents with acute symptoms suggestive of allergies on the ward. What should you do first?

(A) Resolve the symptoms.

(B) Investigate the patient's history of allergies.

(C) Identify triggers and eliminate them.

(D) All of the above.

34. When are ergonomic principles not needed?

(A) When you help patients maintain a comfortable position to receive health care. This could be lying down, sitting down or standing.

(B) When you help patients on operating tables.

(C) When you choose the right assistive device for each patient's needs.

(D) None of the above.

35. General principles for handling biohazardous waste in health care include all of the following except:

(A) Wash hands rigorously after handling any biohazardous material.

(B) Properly dispose of biohazardous material in accordance with stipulated national, state, and local laws.

(C) Design the right procedures to ensure proper disposal of each kind of waste.

(D) None of the above.

36. What is the nurse's role in the demonstration of safe handling techniques to staff and clients?

(A) Mentor.

(B) Educator.

(C) Supervisor.

(D) All of the above.

37. Which of the following is not a major way to ensure safety during radiation therapy?

(A) Time – Minimize exposure time.

(B) Distance – Ensure that there is a safe distance.

(C) Referral – Refer the patient for advanced therapy.

(D) Shielding – Use shielding.

38. A 52-year-old man was brought into the ER unconscious. BP was 220/100 mmhg. He is a known hypertensive, but the patient's relatives say he had not been taking his medication for about two weeks. What kind of variance is this?

(A) Practitioner variance.

(B) System variance.

(C) Patient variance.

(D) None of the above.

39. Examples of home modifications do not include:

(A) Slip-proof floors.

(B) Oxygen provisions.

(C) Emergency exits.

(D) Home CT.

40. One way to educate clients on safety issues is to use:

(A) Teaching aids.

(B) Written instructions.

(C) Presentations.

(D) All of the above.

41. Why are near-misses underreported in health facilities?

(A) No one notices the error.

(B) There is improper documentation.

(C) Staff are penalized for reporting them.

(D) A and C.

42. When there are out-of-place behaviors at the workplace, what should be done?

(A) Report.

(B) Intervene.

(C) Escalate.

(D) All of the above.

43. A patient is supposed to use supportive equipment to move around. He asks you for help in learning to use it. But you have not mastered how to use it well. What do you do?

(A) Teach the patient what you know.

(B) Let the patient know you cannot handle the equipment properly.

(C) Have someone trained in the equipment teach the patient.

(D) B and C.

44. A patient fell after using a pair of crutches that were defective. How could this have been prevented?

(A) The crutches should have been labeled as not for use.

(B) The crutches should have been returned to the manufacturer.

(C) The client should have been more observant.

(D) None of the above.

45. What type of precautions are taken in delivering care to an infectious disease patient?

(A) Standard precautions.

(B) Transmission-based precautions.

(C) PPE.

(D) All of the above.

46. Which of the following actions performed by an intern nurse are unacceptable when providing assistance for a surgical procedure?

(A) Hands placed on the chest after scrubbing.

(B) Focus on the sterile field.

(C) Rearrangement of the sterile field.

(D) Hands dropped after scrubbing.

47. Which of the following is abnormal in a newborn?

(A) Depressed fontanelles.

(B) Blood from the vagina in females.

(C) Labia swelling in females.

(D) All of the above.

48. Sarah is 30 years old. What is a concern she is unlikely to have?

(A) Finding purpose in life.

(B) Learning coping mechanisms.

(C) Exercising to prevent chronic diseases.

(D) Preventing self-consciousness.

49. A previously normotensive woman has an elevated blood pressure of 180/120 mmhg and 170/110 mmhg six hours later. She is eight months pregnant and her urinalysis showed +++ proteins. What is the likely diagnosis and treatment if her BP is uncontrolled?

(A) Diabetes type 2, insulin.

(B) Severe preeclampsia, cesarean section.

(C) Mild preeclampsia, bed rest.

(D) Eclampsia, bed rest.

50. Which of the following should not be done or given to a woman with postpartum hemorrhage who is a known hypertensive?

(A) Oxytocin.

(B) Ergometrine.

(C) Manual exploration of the uterus.

(D) Uterine packing.

51. To confirm a diagnosis of diabetes mellitus after an elevated random blood sugar draw, which of the following tests should not be used?

(A) CBC.

(B) FBS.

(C) HBA1C.

(D) FLP.

52. A woman who looks overweight has come to the clinic because she has some pain in her knees whenever she moves them. From her history, she has a sedentary lifestyle. What investigation/examination is the least important in managing this patient?

(A) BMI.

(B) Knee X-ray.

(C) FLP.

(D) RBS.

53. A man still under anesthesia after surgery lacks readiness to learn in which area?

(A) Physical.

(B) Mental.

(C) Experiential.

(D) All of the above.

54. A study carried out in your community showed that 40% of the population is obese. What can you, as a nurse, do about this?

(A) More research.

(B) Counsel patients.

(C) Provide community health education.

(D) All of the above.

55. Which of these lifestyle choices should patients be counseled against?

(A) Alcoholism.

(B) Substance abuse.

(C) Smoking.

(D) All of the above.

56. Which is the least effective contraceptive method?

(A) Barrier.

(B) Abstinence.

(C) Pills.

(D) Withdrawal.

57. A 37-year-old woman who smokes wants to get contraceptives. Which method is not contraindicated for her?

(A) Vaginal rings.

(B) Diaphragm.

(C) Transdermal patches.

(D) COCP.

58. Which of the following is not true of homeopathic remedies?

(A) They involve a natural approach to treating sickness.

(B) All homeopathic remedies are effective.

(C) The FDA has declared them safe.

(D) None of the above.

59. What is an important first step for a man who has lost his right arm?

(A) Identification with the new state.

(B) Family support.

(C) Assistance with movement.

(D) All of the above.

60. What are the things to assess in a patient who is being managed for bipolar disorder?

(A) Insight.

(B) Frequency of manic episodes.

(C) Adherence to medications.

(D) All of the above.

61. A nurse does not give the prescribed medications to one of her patients on the ward. This is discovered in the following shift. What action was displayed by the first nurse?

(A) Exploitation.

(B) Physical abuse.

(C) Neglect.

(D) Emotional abuse.

62. A woman presented to the ER with her daughter. The five-year-old girl has some injuries on her right arm and a cut on her face. The mother says her daughter fell down at school, but you observe she is very nervous whenever her mom is around. She cannot look up. What do you do?

(A) Ask the mother to wait outside and ask the child a few questions.

(B) Continue treatment and management.

(C) Call social services.

(D) A and C.

63. A 45-year-old man has become hostile and abusive to everyone at home, including his wife and two kids. He no longer speaks to them. He only yells curse words at them at the slightest provocation and has been physically abusive to his kids on two occasions. What are some of the risk factors for his behavior?

(A) Substance abuse.

(B) Crisis at work.

(C) History of being abused when younger.

(D) All of the above.

64. Which of the following statements is false about a nine-year-old girl who was removed from the custody of her abusive uncle?

(A) Intervention means taking the girl from the custody of the abuser.

(B) A nurse must have an open and trusting relationship with the girl.

(C) The girl's care plan will only involve pediatricians.

(D) None of the above.

65. One of the female patients on your ward begins to yell at other patients, which constitutes a nuisance. She also makes threats to assault another patient. What do you do?

(A) Initiate prompt de-escalation.

(B) Suggest stress and relaxation techniques.

(C) Use restraints.

(D) All of the above.

66. A 35-year-old athlete said on TV that he only began to excel in sports because his teacher told him he would never make a great scientist. What type of coping mechanism was employed here?

(A) Dissociation.

(B) Compensation.

(C) Regression.

(D) Sublimation.

67. A 39-year-old woman recently had a messy divorce settled. Her husband got full custody of her kids. She has resorted to cutting herself and hurling obscenities at others. In what level of crisis is this woman?

(A) Level 1.

(B) Level 2.

(C) Level 3.

(D) Level 4.

68. One of your patients does not have the will to live. She has accepted her lot and says she is ready to die because that is what fate has brought her way. What questions should you ask?

(A) What are your family values?

(B) Where is your family?

(C) What makes you feel down?

(D) All of the above.

69. How can you help Dan see that his whole family should participate in family therapy, and not just his son, who is having a hard time bonding with the rest of them?

(A) Tell him if one family member is affected, all are affected.

(B) Tell him his son is not the problem.

(C) Tell him family therapy will help their bonding process.

(D) All of the above.

70. What type of grieving is exhibited when family members begin to feel sad when one of them has a terminal illness but is still alive?

(A) Collective grief.

(B) Cumulative grief.

(C) Anticipatory grief.

(D) Dysfunctional grief.

71. What is the tool used to assess anxiety disorders?

(A) Yale-Brown Obsessive-Compulsive Scale.

(B) Hamilton Rating Scale.

(C) Modified Spielberg State Anxiety Scale.

(D) All of the above.

72. Levi works remotely and was recently discharged from the hospital, where he was managed for hypertension and obesity. What is the implication of his job for the delivery of care?

(A) He must have fixed times when he gets up to take a walk intentionally.

(B) He must register at a gym close to his house.

(C) He must set alarms for his medications.

(D) All of the above.

73. Mia has been making remarkable changes in stress management. How can this be assessed?

(A) She's having fewer panic attacks.

(B) She's showing better judgment.

(C) She has lost weight.

(D) None of the above.

74. "If I understand you correctly, you said he hit you several times with a belt on your back. Is that correct?" What technique of therapeutic communication is this?

(A) Clarification.

(B) Active listening.

(C) Open-ended questions.

(D) Focusing.

75. Which is not a component of a therapeutic environment?

(A) Rules.

(B) Consistency.

(C) Healthy competition.

(D) Boundaries.

76. As the nurse on duty, you noticed that a patient has diarrhea. Which of the following is the best next line of action of care?

(A) Reassure the patient that it is nothing.

(B) Encourage increased intake of meals.

(C) Massage the patient's abdomen.

(D) Commence oral rehydration solution.

77. A patient had a cut on his little finger about four days ago while trimming his flower hedges. The cut seemed to have healed up, but his finger is now swollen, tender and reddish, indicating an abscess. Which of the following is the best next line of care for this patient?

(A) Prescribe antibiotics and analgesics.

(B) Incise and drain the abscess.

(C) Dress the wound with povidone-iodine.

(D) Reassure the patient that the wound will swiftly resolve.

78. A patient had a urethral catheter passed a day ago due to acute urine retention. Retention was relieved and the patient was stable. During your shift as a nurse, the patient reports discomfort and urgency. What is the best next line of action?

(A) Increase intravenous fluid infusion rate.

(B) Start empirical antibiotics immediately.

(C) Prescribe analgesics.

(D) Ensure proper catheter placement and securement.

79. A patient who is paraplegic following a road traffic accident is noticed to have a sore over the sacral and gluteal region. Which of the following is not an appropriate treatment or method of prevention for this patient?

(A) Encourage regular turning in bed.

(B) Extensive debridement of the wound.

(C) Use of a waterbed.

(D) Dress the wound and apply zinc oxide ointment.

80. A patient had a laparotomy for splenectomy following a major splenic rupture after an accident and is currently in recovery. Now the patient complains of pain around the surgical site. Which of the following is the best next line of care?

(A) Elevate the bed to a cardiac position.

(B) Administer prescribed pain medication.

(C) Reassure the patient that the pain will resolve spontaneously.

(D) Open the dressing and examine the surgical site.

81. Regular physiotherapy and outdoor exercise were recommended for a patient who is in the process of recovery from a partial stroke. Which strategy is recommended for this patient?

(A) Eat a heavy meal before exercise.

(B) Use pain medications before exercise.

(C) Skip exercising if exercise.

(D) Warm up before exercise.

82. A patient had a fracture of the left leg following a fall from height and was rushed to the emergency room. Which procedure should be carried out to prevent complications and provide maximum comfort for this patient?

(A) Immobilize the limb and provide analgesia.

(B) Commence active full range of motion exercises.

(C) Lift the limb up above the heart level.

(D) Sedate the patient.

83. A 60-year-old patient had an amputation of the right leg due to extensive diabetic gangrene. Post-surgery, the patient still perceives the limb is present. What is the most appropriate assessment as the nurse on duty?

(A) Psychosis.

(B) Phantom limb experience.

(C) Dementia.

(D) Delirium.

84. A 50-year-old patient who is being managed for type 2 diabetes mellitus is to be evaluated for nutritional assessment. Which of the following is not a component or a needed parameter for the assessment of this patient?

(A) Height.

(B) Weight.

(C) Mid-arm circumference.

(D) Waist circumference.

85. A patient died shortly after being brought to the emergency room following a massive hemorrhage after a car accident. Which of the following is not a component of postmortem care?

(A) Gastric and bladder decompression.

(B) Clean and properly align the body.

(C) Eyes and mouth are closed.

(D) Removal of medical equipment.

86. A patient is on total nasogastric tube feeding due to early-stage corrosive esophagitis. What is the best position to feed this patient?

(A) Recumbent position.

(B) 15 degrees head up.

(C) 30 degrees head up.

(D) 45 degrees head up.

87. A patient who is being managed in your ward complains of insomnia. The patient has no previous history of insomnia. Which of the following is not an appropriate treatment for this patient?

(A) Review of medications for possible drugs that alter sleep pattern.

(B) Commence sedation of the patient.

(C) Counsel the patient on sleep hygiene.

(D) Reduce visitors on the ward.

88. As the nurse on duty, you take an informed consent for a patient who is going to undergo conscious sedation for a minor procedure. The patient asks what the aim of this particular type of anesthesia is compared with other types. What is your most appropriate response?

(A) Tell him it is to provide relaxation and an anxiolytic state while maintaining consciousness.

(B) Tell him it is to provide total relief from pain during the procedure.

(C) Tell him it is to cause a state of deep sleep and unconsciousness.

(D) Tell him it is to minimize post-op pain.

89. An 88-year-old male patient being given palliative treatment for advanced-stage lung cancer complains of pain despite being on opioid medication such as morphine. What is the best next line of care?

(A) Increase the dose of morphine after the maximum safe dose.

(B) Reassure the patient.

(C) Use other nonpharmacological/adjunct treatment.

(D) Sedate the patient.

90. A patient who has been on intravenous therapy via peripherally placed venous access is to be administered an intravenous medication. Which of the following is the most appropriate to ensure safe administration of the medication?

(A) Assess the patient's vital signs before administration of the medication.

(B) Give the medication as quickly as possible.

(C) Use the widest-bore IV cannula to administer the medication.

(D) Check the IV site for signs of infiltration and infection.

91. As the nurse administering a medication, you read the drug leaflet and note that the drug has a high rate of first metabolism. Which drug is this likely to be?

(A) Glyburide.

(B) Diazepam.

(C) Acetaminophen.

(D) Vitamin C.

92. You are discharging a patient with a nicotine patch to manage cigarette addiction. What route of drug administration is employed by this medication?

(A) Transdermal.

(B) Enteral.

(C) Subcutaneous.

(D) Sublingual.

93. A patient being managed for type 2 diabetes mellitus is being counseled on self-insulin injection therapy at home. Which of the following is not essential counseling information?

(A) Daily weight check.

(B) Ensure check of random blood glucose before administration.

(C) Identification of symptoms of hypoglycemia such as diaphoresis, dizziness, blurred vision, etc.

(D) Rotation of injection site of insulin.

94. A pediatric patient is brought to the emergency room convulsing after being involved in a fire. He has extensive burns over his upper and lower limbs. What is the most appropriate route for administering anticonvulsants?

(A) Sublingual.

(B) Subcutaneous.

(C) Intramuscular.

(D) Rectal.

95. A patient being treated for bacterial peritonitis was placed on intravenous Amikacin 180 mg daily. The vial comes in 500 mg preparation in 5 mls. How many mls should you administer?

(A) 0.6 mls.

(B) 1.2 mls.

(C) 1.8 mls.

(D) 2.2 mls.

96. A patient is being transfused due to post-anemia following elective surgery. Which of the following changes in vital signs is usually the first indication of a transfusion reaction?

(A) Increase in blood pressure.

(B) Increase in respiration.

(C) Decrease in heart rate.

(D) Increase in temperature.

97. A 14-year-old boy who is a known asthmatic was brought to the pediatric emergency due to difficulty breathing. He was commenced on nebulized salbutamol therapy. What is a common side effect of this therapy?

(A) Bradypnea.

(B) Tachycardia.

(C) Diaphoresis.

(D) Excessive salivation.

98. What complications can a lower limb peripheral intravenous catheter cause?

(A) Mastitis and phlebitis.

(B) Phlebitis and embolism.

(C) Pain and diabetic foot.

(D) All of the above.

99. When do you know you are in the vein during peripheral IV cannulations?

(A) 45 degrees.

(B) 60 degrees.

(C) When there is a flashback.

(D) 30–60 degrees.

100. Which of the following statements about venous access methods is false?

(A) A central and peripheral venous access device can be used for venous access.

(B) Peripheral intravenous devices are utilized for short-term intravenous therapy.

(C) The distal veins on the dominant hand are the ideal choice.

(D) The patient's mastectomy side is not used.

101. Which of the following patients must be trained in administering their own subcutaneous injections?

(A) HIV/AIDS patients.

(B) Obese patients.

(C) Diabetic patients.

(D) All of the above.

102. To determine the accuracy of medication orders for clients, what things should be observed?

(A) Completion of the medical order.

(B) Accuracy of the order.

(C) Client allergies.

(D) All of the above.

103. What are the major advantages of intravenous medications?

(A) 100% bioavailability and swift onset of action.

(B) Swift allergic reactions and hypersensitivities.

(C) Infections.

(D) Requires technical skill to set up.

104. Which of the following is not a route for drug administration?

(A) Transdermal.

(B) Inhalation.

(C) Topical.

(D) None of the above.

105. What is an example of a drug that can only be administered via the intravenous route?

(A) Cisplatin.

(B) Amoxicillin.

(C) Cefuroxime.

(D) All of the above.

106. In an emergency involving a Para 5 woman who is currently having a postpartum hemorrhage, what kind of cannula should you opt for in setting an intravenous line?

(A) 14g, 16g.

(B) 22g, 24g.

(C) 20g, 24g.

(D) 18g, 24g.

107. Nitroglycerin is administered through what route in angina?

(A) Oral.

(B) Transdermal.

(C) Sublingual.

(D) Intravenous.

108. Which of the following are not important in illness management?

(A) Treatable signs and symptoms of chronic diseases.

(B) Treatment procedures.

(C) Financial cost.

(D) None of the above.

109. What are the loading and maintenance doses for the Zuspan regimen in the management of preeclampsia?

(A) 4 g Mgso4—2 g Mgso4 per hour over 24 hrs.

(B) 14 g Mgso4, 2 g hydralazine.

(C) 4 g Mgso4—1 g Mgso4 per hour over 24 hrs.

(D) 14 g Mgso4—2 g Mgso4 per hour over 24 hrs.

110. What are the loading and maintenance doses for the Pritchard regimen in the management of preeclampsia?

(A) 4g Mgso4—2g Mgso4 per hour over 24 hrs.

(B) 14 g Mgso4—5 g Mgso4 4 hrly.

(C) 4 g Mgso4—1 g Mgso4 per hour over 24 hrs.

(D) 14 g Mgso4—2 g Mgso4 per hour over 24 hrs.

111. How is adrenaline given in CPR?

(A) 2 mg IV bolus every minute.

(B) 1 mg IV bolus every 5 minutes.

(C) 5 mg IV bolus every minute.

(D) 10 mg IV bolus every 1 minute.

112. How would you manage a child brought in with seizures at the ER?

(A) Administer anticonvulsants.

(B) Position the child on the left side of his body.

(C) Suction as necessary.

(D) All of the above.

113. A 25-year-old female presents to the ER with an elevated blood pressure of 190/110 mmhg, weakness, and facial puffiness, which regresses as the day goes by. What are your differentials?

(A) Hypertension.

(B) Chronic kidney disease.

(C) Cancer.

(D) All of the above.

114. A 45-year-old man comes into the ER complaining of fatigue. His pulse rate is 90 bpm, irregular. Heart rate is 120 bpm; other vitals are stable. What is your differential?

(A) Asystole.

(B) CKD.

(C) Atrial fibrillation.

(D) Ventriculoseptal defect.

115. A 25-year-old man presents to the clinic with a respiratory rate of 36 cpm, with chest tightness, wheezing, and difficulty breathing. What is the likely diagnosis and first line of management?

(A) Tuberculosis—place on oxygen.

(B) Congestive cardiac failure—IV furosemide.

(C) Asthma—nebulize.

(D) Any of the above.

116. Which of the following is a major indication for a random blood glucose test?

(A) Unconscious patient.

(B) Dehydrated patient with ketone breath.

(C) Sickle cell patient.

(D) A and B.

117. All of the following are ECG findings for a patient with myocardial infarction except:

(A) ST-segment elevation.

(B) T wave inversion.

(C) ST-segment depression.

(D) None of the above.

118. What is the most important thing a nurse must do before proceeding with any test on a client?

(A) Get materials ready.

(B) Position the patient.

(C) Get informed consent.

(D) All of the above.

119. Which of the following tests do not require blood withdrawal?

(A) CBC.

(B) EUCR.

(C) LFT.

(D) Mantoux test.

120. What is the 24-hour urine sample collection mostly used for?

(A) To measure 24-hour glucose.

(B) To measure 24-hour protein.

(C) To measure 24-hour WBC.

(D) None of the above.

121. How would you prevent a 24-year-old man from going into shock after being in a car accident and bleeding profusely?

(A) Stop bleeding.

(B) Use volume expanders.

(C) Get blood for a transfusion.

(D) All of the above.

122. A 70-year-old female patient presents with delayed healing of a wound on the lower third of the leg. The patient has not been eating well for the last month. How should you counsel the patient?

(A) Tell her that poor diet is a risk factor for delayed wound healing.

(B) Counsel the patient on wound care.

(C) A and B.

(D) Counsel the patient on diabetes and its effect on wound healing.

123. What should you do if the venipuncture site for a patient does not stop bleeding?

(A) Apply pressure with your thumb and gauze for three to five minutes.

(B) Admit the patient.

(C) Call for help if bleeding continues for more than eight minutes.

(D) A and C.

124. A 30-year-old patient presents at night with a blood pressure of 80/50 mmhg, weakness, and almost falls when she trics to stand. What is your next line of action?

(A) Set up isotonic IV fluids.

(B) Do a fasting blood glucose test.

(C) Take samples for baseline investigations while setting the line.

(D) A and C.

125. Which of the following is not considered a major risk of orthopedic implant surgery?

(A) Osteomyelitis.

(B) Dislodgement.

(C) Pain.

(D) None of the above.

126. What are some signs of surgical site infection?

(A) Offensive odor from the wound site.

(B) Pus from the wound.

(C) Fever.

(D) All of the above.

127. A patient cannot move one side of his face when he smiles. What is the likely diagnosis and what nerve is most likely affected?

(A) Bell's Palsy, CN VII.

(B) Influenza, CN XII.

(C) Paralysis, CN X.

(D) Stroke, CN VII.

128. What therapeutic agent is commonly implicated in hypoglycemia?

(A) Glucose.

(B) Insulin.

(C) Sugar.

(D) Normal saline.

129. What is the role of the nurse for a patient who will be put under general anesthesia?

(A) Educate and reassure the patient.

(B) Anesthetize the patient.

(C) Obtain informed consent.

(D) A and C.

130. One common complication of spinal anesthesia is:

(A) Back pain.

(B) Headaches.

(C) Confusion.

(D) All of the above.

131. One major complication of long-standing hypertension is:

(A) Ventricular hypertrophy.

(B) Atrial hypertrophy.

(C) Atrial fibrillation.

(D) All of the above.

132. Accumulation of waste products in the blood is an indicator of likely damage or injury to the:

(A) Liver.

(B) Kidneys.

(C) Heart.

(D) Lungs.

133. What is the most worrisome complication of hyperbilirubinemia in neonates?

(A) Kernicterus.

(B) Bronze baby syndrome.

(C) Opisthotonus.

(D) All of the above.

134. How does phototherapy treat jaundice?

(A) It breaks down the bilirubin into soluble isomers.

(B) It breaks down bilirubin into insoluble isomers.

(C) Isomers are excreted in the urine.

(D) A and C.

135. Which of the following is not an indication of central line placement?

(A) Difficult peripheral access in an emergency.

(B) High volume/flow procedures.

(C) Placement of vena cava filter.

(D) Skin infection.

136. What are the contraindications of a core needle biopsy?

(A) Uncooperative patients/uncontrollable movements.

(B) Uncorrectable bleeding disorder.

(C) No safe path for the needle.

(D) All of the above.

137. Which of the following is not involved in suctioning?

(A) Preoxygenation.

(B) Lubrication of suction catheter tip.

(C) Advancing the catheter tip into the airways.

(D) Post-oxygenation.

138. Which of the following materials are not needed for wound dressing?

(A) Sterile gauze.

(B) Bandage.

(C) Normal saline.

(D) Needle holder.

139. Providing pulmonary hygiene does not involve:

(A) Postural hygiene.

(B) Deep breathing.

(C) Percussion.

(D) Auscultation.

140. Where is the most common site for an AV fistula?

(A) Forearm/upper arm.

(B) Thigh.

(C) Chest.

(D) Neck.

141. A 55-year-old man presents to the ER with shortness of breath and swollen feet. He is a known hypertensive. BP = 170/90 mmhg; SPO2 = 78% IRA. What is your first line of action?

(A) Administer IV Furosemide.

(B) Place on oxygen.

(C) Monitor vitals.

(D) Take samples for investigation.

142. A woman presents at the ER with a blood pressure of 85/65 mmhg. She falls when she tries to get up. Her lips are dry. What is the next line of action?

(A) Run CBC, EUCR, LFT.

(B) Set up IV ringer's lactate.

(C) Commence blood transfusion.

(D) All of the above.

143. What is the characteristic ECG feature of hyperkalemia?

(A) ST-segment elevation.

(B) Shortened PR interval.

(C) Tall Tented T waves.

(D) Increased P-wave amplitude.

144. How would you recognize a pacemaker on an ECG?

(A) Pacemaker ST depression.

(B) Pacemaker spikes.

(C) T-wave depression.

(D) Widened QRS complex.

145. Which is not a contraindication for a pacing device?

(A) Nonrecurring AV block.

(B) Asymptomatic first-degree AV block.

(C) Asymptomatic second-degree Mobitz block type I.

(D) Sinus node dysfunction.

146. Which is not an indication for a pacemaker?

(A) Acquired AV block.

(B) Alternating bundle branch block.

(C) Unresolving, symptomatic bradycardia.

(D) Asymptomatic bradycardia while sleeping.

147. A patient had a pacemaker inserted recently. Within the first six months, what is your most serious concern?

(A) Device-related complications.

(B) Hematoma formation.

(C) Pneumothorax.

(D) Infections.

148. What are the most important things a client must be educated about in illness management?

(A) Etiology.

(B) Treatment.

(C) Pathophysiology.

(D) All of the above.

149. What test is the most important in the diagnosis of asthma?

(A) Lung compliance.

(B) Pulse oximetry.

(C) Spirometry.

(D) All of the above.

150. Which of the following statements is false?

(A) An acute condition is a sudden, rapid health condition that requires an emergency response.

(B) A chronic condition is a long-standing condition.

(C) A subacute condition is the same as an acute condition.

(D) A recurrent condition occurs repeatedly, often with a resolution in between episodes.

Test 4: Answers and Explanations

1. (D) A and B.

In such a situation, the nurse should confirm that the patient has been taking the medication according to the prescription of the physician. If this has been done, then the physicians should be informed.

2. (B) Let her healthcare proxy decide.

A living will is a document that usually contains a list of the types of treatments and health care interventions that an individual does or does not want when they can no longer give informed consent. Since the procedure to be done was not included in Mrs. Parker's living will, the responsibility falls to the healthcare proxy to decide who makes the decision.

3. (C) Right to reject advance directives.

The right to reject advance directives is not included in the Self-Determination Act. The Self-Determination Act only gives the patient the right to either accept or reject care on admission to any healthcare facility. This act also gives patients the right to *ask* for advance directives.

4. (D) None of the above.

All the options listed are involved in advocacy. Advocacy involves being present and listening to patients, which would involve observing both verbal and nonverbal cues, discussing specific treatment modalities with clients and advocating for staff members.

5. (D) None of the above.

The discussion of specified treatment modalities includes the treatment itself, the procedure, benefits, possible risks and side effects, the personnel carrying out the procedure, and other alternatives to the procedure.

6. (B) 5.

The American Nurses Association has created the five Rights of Delegation to help in the appropriate delegation of responsibilities. The five rights are the right person, the right task, the right circumstances, the right direction/communication, and the right supervision/evaluation.

7. (B) What is the state of the patient?

For the right circumstance, healthcare personnel should ask if the patient is stable or unstable. Care of a stable patient can be delegated to others. Only a registered nurse should handle the care of an unstable patient.

8. (B) Some tasks for this patient can be delegated.

From the vitals that have been given, this patient is unstable. Therefore, not all tasks can be delegated for this patient. Some tasks involve client needs that follow set routines and require lower levels of professional judgment and competence. Such tasks can be easily delegated. However, since this patient is unstable, there can be rapid changes that require tasks that involve quick judgment calls and higher competence. Such tasks should not be delegated.

9. (D) Circulatory, airway, breathing.

The framework highlighted here is the ABCs of resuscitation. The ABCs of resuscitation are airway, breathing, and cardiovascular or circulatory system. This is useful in deciding where to start attending to a patient who has undergone a cardiac arrest. It is important to note that the recent update has changed the sequence to CAB, meaning chest compressions come first, followed by airway and then breathing.

10. (D) B and C.

Transferring a patient involves moving the patient to another level of care. When this happens, nurses are expected to coordinate the process. They ensure that every patient is treated at the right level of care. They also educate the clients and their families on when this needs to be done and give the reasons, the modalities, and the outcomes they are trying to achieve or prevent. They also update the patient's plan of care.

11. (A) HIPAA.

HIPAA stands for Health Insurance Portability and Accountability Act. It protects the personal information of the client, e.g., name, date of birth, social security number, diagnosis, and treatment. This act ensures that only those involved in the management or care of the patient have access to the information.

12. (B) Informed consent.

Informed consent means that patients have the right to know all available treatment options and decide which they prefer. Informed consent also means that patients should be clearly informed about their condition and the proposed treatment, including the benefits, risks, side effects, recovery, and any other information about the procedure.

13. (D) All of the above.

Nurses must know the most important things to look out for in a patient's condition. The vital signs provide a general indicator of the vital organs in the body. The mood gives an idea about the mental status of the patient. Adverse drug events must be reported so that they are not repeated. Nurses must channel this information to the appropriate healthcare personnel for immediate action.

14. (D) A and B.

Licensed practical nurses are licensed health care professionals. They can perform both sterile and non-sterile procedures, including collection of specimens. Patient care technicians are non-licensed assistants who help nurses to provide direct and indirect care. They also help perform non-sterile procedures requiring little technical expertise, such as collecting specimens, documenting vital signs, and assisting with patient movement and exercises and other patient activities required for daily living. Nursing supervisors are responsible for patient supervision and receive reports from several nurses under their supervision.

15. (D) Social workers.

Social workers are primarily involved in ensuring that the patient is appropriately moved in the continuum of care and there is no deficit after the patient is discharged. They counsel patients and can also provide psychological support. They are essential in cases of child abuse, neglect, or malpractice and can provide much-needed support for victims.

16. (D) None of the above.

The nursing process includes planning, assessing, implementing, and evaluating.

17. (D) Suggest a compromise.

Compromise or negotiation is a healthy way of resolving conflicts, as both parties must make a move to meet in the middle. It emphasizes a focus on common goals and interests, which in this setting should be the delivery of quality care rather than focusing on personal interests and desires. All other options listed are unhelpful in resolving conflict.

18. (A) Indirect.

HIPAA restricts patient information to only those who need to know. This need-to-know population is divided into two groups: those who render direct and indirect patient care. Direct patient care refers to those who directly provide a form of care to the patient, e.g., nurses, physical therapists, doctors, etc. Indirect care covers those who do not directly provide a form of care but still have a role to play in their care, e.g., insurance, directors of nursing, etc.

19. (A) She has violated patient rights according to HIPAA.

The confidentiality that HIPAA mandates healthcare workers to keep is not just limited to written information. It also covers electronic and online information about a patient's health status and must not be shared with those that need to know except when consented to by the patient in writing.

20. (C) Patient, Plan, Purpose, Problems, Precaution.

The 5 Ps in the continuity of care are Patient, Plan, Purpose, Problems and Precautions. These 5 Ps are a system of reporting essential information that must be passed on to the next nurse shift.

21. (D) None of the above.

Management of care involves the provision of nursing care, coordination of nursing care, and health care delivery in such a way that it makes the health care delivery setting safer for both the client and the health care personnel.

22. (A) Prevent illness.

The fundamental responsibility of the nurse is to prevent illness, promote health, restore health, and alleviate suffering.

23. (D) All of the above.

Patients at the end of life have needs that are different from routine patients. They need physical, psychological, spiritual, and physiological care. Some of the physical needs might be adequate nutrition and fluids and pain management. Psychological needs can be diverse. Such patients might battle with confusion, sleep disturbances, or depression. Nurses should educate clients about what to expect at this stage as well as the things to be sorted out, such as legal documents and advance directives. The clients' families and support system should also be educated about what to expect toward the end of life.

24. (A) Verification.

After orders are received, the first thing the nurse is expected to do is to verify them by asking for confirmation or clarity from health care providers. This ensures that there are no errors or omitted actions. Care is then planned or updated.

25. (A) Beneficence.

According to the principle of beneficence, a nurse is expected to act in the best interest of the patient.

26. (B) Risk management.

Risk management is concerned with the reduction and elimination of health care hazards that can result in a liability to the company. Examples of these are infant abduction, patient falls, and medication errors. These risks can be identified and eliminated using root cause analysis. Outcome measures focus on the outcomes of care.

27. (B) Problem definition, measurement, data analysis, improvements, control.

The Six Sigma method involves problem definition, measuring, analysis of data, improvements to make, and control.

28. (D) Self-help groups.

Self-help groups in the community are very helpful for those who battle addiction or other mental health conditions, e.g., schizophrenia.

29. (D) None of the above.

Common allergy symptoms include but are not limited to tachycardia; bradycardia; swelling; numbness, itching or tingling at the exposure point; breathing difficulties; rashes or bumps; hypotension and hypertension. Swelling, numbness, or tingling sensations around the lips, mouth or tongue are usually indications of extremely serious allergic reactions.

30. (D) Hunger.

The frequency of falls is affected by factors like the patient's developmental stage, aging, lifestyle, and mental status. Children in the developmental stages and the elderly are more prone to accidents and injuries than younger adults, while the poor mental status of a patient can make the individual prone to self-imposed injury.

31. (C) Bedside monitors.

Bedside monitors are best for patients in the ICU who might be unconscious and unable to use a call bell or verbally express their needs.

32. (C) A and B.

To avoid mismatched prescriptions and wrong medications, patients must be properly identified and the order verified. It is recommended to have at least two distinct identifiers aside from the room number of clients. Room numbers, in themselves, should not be used as unique identifiers. Nurses should consider using patients' full names, complete dates of birth, and some other unique identification codes.

33. (A) Resolve the symptoms.

Indications of extremely serious allergic reactions include swelling, numbness, or tingling sensations around the lips, mouth, or tongue. The first thing is to address the emergency before taking a history. Triggers can be identified from the history and then eliminated.

34. (D) None of the above.

Ergonomic principles should be observed when you move patients from one point to the other on stretchers, wheelchairs and so on, to help patients maintain a comfortable position to receive health care. This could be lying down, sitting down or standing. They should also be observed when you help patients on operating tables or choose the right assistive device for each patient's needs and providing therapy.

35. (D) None of the above.

All the options are part of the general principles for handling biohazardous waste.

36. (B) Educator.

When the nurse demonstrates safe handling techniques to staff and clients, they assume the role of an educator. In such situations, the nurse may be required to demonstrate how to safely handle hazardous substances to other staff members, as well as to clients.

37. (C) Referral – Refer the patient for advanced therapy.

Radiation safety is generally about three key principles. Time: Minimize the duration of exposure and reduce the dose of radiation. Distance: The farther one is from the radiation source, the less radiation they will receive. Shielding: Use barriers like lead aprons to protect the patient against radiation.

38. (C) Patient variance.

Patient variance is an irregular occurrence associated with excesses on the part of the client. In this question, this patient has likely developed complications because he did not comply with the treatment.

39. (D) Home CT.

Home modifications are solutions that provide an enabling home environment for clients. Factors like lighting, handrails, slip-proof floors, oxygen, and emergency exits are crucial to the improvement of the patient's well-being and ability to adjust their lifestyles to the new health conditions they may be managing. Home CT is not an essential part of modifications.

40. (D) All of the above.

Different formats can be used to educate clients on safety issues. Clients may be presented with written instructions or other teaching aids that will aid retention and also serve as a handy resource they can always return to.

41. (D) A and C.

Errors and near misses remain under-reported in healthcare facilities due to various factors, such as fear of penalization, overlooked errors, and ignorance of how to document such errors.

42. (D) All of the above.

Registered nurses are required to report, intervene and/or de-escalate unsafe practices of health care personnel. RNs are responsible to look out for other healthcare workers and report out-of-place behaviors and unsafe practices that could pose threats to clients and other persons in the healthcare environment. Such unsafe practices include substance abuse, improper care, biases directed toward certain clients, etc.

43. (D) B and C.

Clients should be trained on how to safely handle equipment, particularly any they will be using at home, away from staff members' oversight. When you are not sure about how to use equipment, explain this to the patient and get a professional to teach them.

44. (A) The crutches should have been labeled as not for use.

Labels allow everyone to know that equipment is not suitable for use.

45. (B) Transmission-based precautions.

Transmission-based precautions are preventive and infection control measures that are utilized to combat and inhibit the spread of specific infections. These precautionary procedures are informed based on the type of infection and its medium of transmission. For infectious diseases, which are spread by droplets and contact, the precautions would be based on the routes.

46. (D) Hands dropped after scrubbing.

The nurse must never drop her hands below the sterile field after scrubbing. Only sterile items should be placed on the sterile field. The nurse should never have the sterile field below the waist level and should not lean over or turn their back to the sterile field. A cough or sneeze over the sterile field contaminates it.

47. (A) Depressed fontanelles.

Depressed fontanelles can be a sign of reduced intracranial pressure, which can be due to dehydration. Normal fontanelles should be soft and fat, with no depression or bulge. A bulge can be a sign of raised intracranial depression. Some females may have some level of swelling in the labia and blood from the vagina.

48. (D) Preventing self-consciousness.

Sarah is a young adult in the intimacy vs. isolation stage. Typical expectations are seeking purpose in life; the development of healthy coping mechanisms to deal with the demands of work, relationships, and other commitments; and preventive steps to reduce the occurrence of chronic conditions with age. Self-consciousness is more characteristic of adolescents.

49. (B) Severe preeclampsia, cesarean section.

Severe preeclampsia is defined as blood pressure greater than or equal to 160/10 mmhg on at least two occasions six hours apart, protein of 3+ or more. Treatment is delivery of the fetus since blood pressure remains uncontrolled.

50. (B) Ergometrine.

Ergometrine is known to increase blood pressure. It could cause complications in a known hypertensive.

51. (A) CBC.

A complete blood count is not relatively significant in the diagnosis of diabetes mellitus. The fasting blood sugar (FBS) is essential; the HBA1C helps to see the blood glucose profile over a long time and the FLP usually shows some derangement which increases the risks of cardiovascular diseases in type 2 diabetes mellitus.

52. (D) RBS.

BMI helps to confirm if the patient is overweight or obese, which is a risk factor for knee pain. A knee X-ray helps to show what is going on in the knee, most likely arthritis. FLP helps to show the lipid profile.

53. (A) Physical.

A man that is under the effects of anesthesia might still be unconscious or drowsy. He is physically not capable of learning at that point. Physical readiness involves the measures of ability, the complexity of the task, the effect of the environment, the health status of the individual and even gender. The measures of physical ability determine if a patient is ready to learn or not.

54. (D) All of the above.

The nurse must be ready to educate people and carry out more research to improve health care delivery and outcomes around their environment. Community health education refers to the study and development of health characteristics among target populations. From time to time, nurses must provide education to help achieve these objectives of developing health characteristics. When needs are identified, the nurse can devise a plan to intervene as needed. It might involve educating community members via oral presentations, counseling and guidance.

55. (D) All of the above.

Nurses should counsel patients against lifestyle choices that predispose them to illness. These include alcoholism, substance abuse, smoking, obesity, sedentary lifestyle, etc.

56. (D) Withdrawal.

The withdrawal method is the least effective of the options given. It involves ejaculating outside the vagina during coitus.

57. (B) Diaphragm.

The major contraindication to diaphragm use is latex sensitivity. Other methods that are listed are contraindicated in a patient that takes cigarettes.

58. (B) All homeopathic remedies are effective.

Not all homeopathic remedies are effective. The FDA only attests to the safety of homeopathy, not the effectiveness of all its remedies.

59. (A) Identification with the new state.

The patient has to first come to accept the new state that he is in, as it will permanently alter his life. Once this is done, then other things can follow, such as family support, assistance with movement, etc.

60. (D) All of the above.

All the things listed must be assessed to determine if care is effective or not. Insight is the ability of this patient to be aware of their mental condition.

61. (C) Neglect.

The nurse exhibited neglect. Neglect refers to the deprivation of basic or essential care needed to help a patient maintain physical or mental health. Neglect can be due to actions or inactions, which include failure to provide food, water, shelter, medications or access to health care.

62. (D) A and C.

The injuries are likely due to physical abuse from the mother. The best thing to do is to ask the woman to stay outside and then to ask the girl some questions. The nurse must be able to establish an open, trusting and nonjudgmental relationship with the girl. Children only open up when they feel safe. Nurses should be skillful at asking questions. Social services should also be involved as the child might need to be separated from the abuser.

63. (D) All of the above.

All the options listed are risk factors for abuse. Others include mental health disorders, physical disability, poor anger management skills, etc.

64. (C) The girl's care plan will only involve pediatricians.

This is false. The girl's care plan will require multidisciplinary management such as social health services, psychologists, counselors, physicians, lab scientists, nutritionists, etc. It will also mean taking her from the custody of the abuser.

65. (C) Use restraints.

The use of restraints is a last resort, but here, the patient can constitute harm to herself or other patients. So, restraints have to be used. A nurse should also quickly inform security whenever she feels that the safety of any patient or personnel on the ward is endangered. Offensive speech with inappropriate behavior should not be condoned at the health facility.

66. (B) Compensation.

Compensation is when a person succeeds in one activity or field in order to compensate for another area of failure. Here the athlete used his excellence in sports to compensate for his failure in science class.

67. (D) Level 4.

At Level 4, the patient begins to feel isolated, detached and completely overwhelmed by life events. Patients might even begin to entertain thoughts and acts of violence toward themselves and others.

68. (D) All of the above.

Family values can influence the way illness and death are perceived. Some believe their health and the outcome of health interventions are fate and might not be so motivated to take steps because they believe it all depends on fate.

69. (D) All of the above.

The nurse must be able to educate Dan and other family members on the need for group therapy and its benefits. Many times all family members are affected to varying degrees, and all play roles that affect each other positively or negatively.

70. (C) Anticipatory grief.

Anticipatory grief is the grief process that begins before the event happens. It is usually seen in cases like terminal illnesses, loss, or amputation of a body part.

71. (D) All of the above.

Tools for assessing anxiety disorders include the Yale-Brown Obsessive-Compulsive Scale, the Modified Spielberger State Anxiety Scale, and the Hamilton Rating Scale for anxiety.

72. (D) All of the above.

If he wants to achieve a good healthcare outcome, Levi must exercise more regularly and take his medications.

73. (B) She's showing better judgment.

Stress management can easily be assessed by observance of Mia's use of stress management techniques. She will show less fear and make better decisions. There will be no negative physiological changes.

74. (A) Clarification.

Clarification is an attempt to understand exactly what the patient said. In clarification, the nurse will usually restate, paraphrase, and reflect on what the patient has said.

75. (C) Healthy competition.

Competition is not a component of a therapeutic environment. Patients in a healthcare setting are not meant to compete with anyone. They are meant to focus on recovery. Some of the elements of a therapeutic environment include rules and boundaries, appropriate behavior, consistency, and client expectations.

76. (D) Commence oral rehydration solution.

Diarrhea can lead to dehydration. The best immediate action for a nurse to take is to initiate oral rehydration to replace lost fluids and electrolytes. While reassuring the patient can be a part of care, it doesn't address the immediate medical need. Encouraging meals may not be advisable without knowing the cause of diarrhea, and massaging the abdomen is not a standard care procedure for diarrhea.

77. (B) Incise and drain the abscess.

An abscess usually requires drainage to release the pus and relieve the symptoms. If you dress the wound with povidone-iodine, it may help prevent infection, but it won't treat an existing abscess. Reassuring the patient without taking action could cause complications.

78. (D) Ensure proper catheter placement and securement.

Discomfort and urgency after catheterization can be due to improper placement or movement of the catheter. The first step is to check its position and make sure it's secure.

79. (B) Extensive debridement of the wound.

Bed sores or pressure ulcers require careful attention, especially in paraplegic patients. Regular turning in bed, the use of specialized beds like waterbeds, and dressing the wound are all measures that are used to treat or prevent pressure ulcers. Extensive debridement without appropriate assessment and indication can be harmful and is not a primary preventive measure.

80. (B) Administer prescribed pain medication.

After surgery, it's common for patients to experience pain at the surgical site. You should administer prescribed pain medication since it is the first step in managing post-operative pain.

81. (D) Warm up before exercise.

Warming up before exercise is important for all individuals, especially those who are recovering from medical conditions like a stroke. It helps prepare the body for more strenuous activities, reduces the risk of injury, and improves the efficacy of the exercise.

82. (A) Immobilize the limb and provide analgesia.

In cases of fractures, it's vital to immobilize the limb to prevent further injury and reduce pain. If you provide pain relief, it will also ensure the patient's comfort.

83. (B) Phantom limb experience.

Many individuals who undergo amputation experience a sensation that the amputated limb is still present. This phenomenon is called a phantom limb experience. It's not indicative of psychosis, dementia, or delirium, but is rather a common neurological occurrence after amputation.

84. (A) Height.

For a nutritional assessment of a type 2 diabetic patient, parameters like weight, mid-arm circumference, and waist circumference are directly linked to nutritional status. These parameters are also related to metabolic health risks that are associated with obesity and insulin resistance.

85. (A) Gastric and bladder decompression.

Postmortem care is used to make the deceased look peaceful and preserve dignity. Clean the body, align it properly, and close the eyes and mouth. Then, remove any medical equipment. Gastric and bladder decompression is not a routine component of postmortem care.

86. (D) 45 degrees head up.

Patients on nasogastric tube feeding should be positioned so that their head is elevated at about 30 to 45 degrees. This reduces the risk of aspiration, which can cause pneumonia. The head position at 45 degrees is known as the semi-Fowler's position and is most commonly recommended for such feedings.

87. (B) Commence sedation of the patient.

You should not sedate a patient for insomnia unless it's critically needed. Before administering sedatives, it's important to review the medications the patient is on, as some can affect sleep. Sleep hygiene counseling can be beneficial. Also, if you reduce the number of visitors, this can also help decrease disturbances and promote sleep.

88. (A) Tell him it is to provide relaxation and an anxiolytic state while maintaining consciousness.

Conscious sedation provides relaxation and reduces anxiety while allowing the patient to remain awake and be able to communicate. It doesn't provide complete pain relief or deep sleep.

89. (C) Use other nonpharmacological/adjunct treatment.

For patients with cancer pain that's not well-controlled with opioids, it's important to consider nonpharmacological treatments or adjunct medications that can help the patient control pain.

90. (D) Check the IV site for signs of infiltration and infection.

Before administering IV medication, it's essential to check the IV site for signs of infiltration (where the IV fluid goes into the surrounding tissue) and infection. This ensures that the medication will be delivered into the vein as intended.

91. (B) Diazepam.

The term "first-pass metabolism" or "first-pass effect" refers to the liver's ability to metabolize drugs before they reach the systemic circulation. Diazepam undergoes significant first-pass metabolism, which reduces the amount of the drug that reaches the systemic circulation after oral administration.

92. (A) Transdermal.

Nicotine patches deliver the medication through the skin directly into the bloodstream. This route of administration is termed "transdermal." It provides a slow, steady release of medication over an extended period.

93. (A) Daily weight check.

The monitoring of weight is not directly related to self-insulin injection therapy. The other options are necessary for someone who is self-administering insulin.

94. (D) Rectal.

In emergency situations where a patient is convulsing and there are challenges with oral, intravenous, or intramuscular routes (e.g., because of extensive burns), the rectal route can be an effective way to deliver anticonvulsants such as diazepam.

95. (C) 1.8 mls.

To determine the amount to administer:

If 500 mg is in 5 mls, then 1 mg will be in 5/500 mls = 0.01 mls.

For 180 mg: 180 mg x 0.01 mls/mg = 1.8 mls.

96. (D) Increase in temperature.

One of the early signs of a transfusion reaction is a fever or an increase in temperature. The patient may also exhibit other symptoms such as chills, back pain, and hemoglobinuria. Immediate cessation of the transfusion and prompt assessment and intervention are vital if a transfusion reaction is suspected.

97. (B) Tachycardia.

Nebulized salbutamol is a beta-2 adrenergic agonist and can cause side effects due to its stimulant effect on the heart. One of the most common side effects is tachycardia or an increased heart rate. This can be accompanied by feelings of palpitations or a racing heart.

98. (B) Phlebitis and embolism.

Peripheral intravenous catheters, especially when placed in the lower limb, can cause complications such as phlebitis (inflammation of the vein) and embolism (obstruction of a blood vessel by a clot or foreign substance). Mastitis is an inflammation of the breast tissue and is unrelated to IV catheters. Diabetic foot is related to complications of diabetes mellitus and is not directly linked to peripheral IV catheters.

99. (C) When there is a flashback.

When inserting a peripheral IV cannula, the appearance of a “flashback” (which is a visible return of blood in the hub or chamber of the cannula) indicates that the needle tip has entered the vein. This is the moment when practitioners know they are in the vein and can then proceed with the cannulation process.

100. (C) The distal veins on the dominant hand are the ideal choice.

The distal veins on the non-dominant hand are the ideal choice so the client can fully use the dominant hand. When patients have accessible and usable veins, peripheral intravenous devices are utilized for short-term intravenous therapy, including fluids, electrolytes, medicines, and chemotherapy. A patient’s mastectomy side, paralyzed side, or side with a dialysis access device are not used.

101. (C) Diabetic patients.

Diabetic patients usually require subcutaneous insulin injections, especially type 1. They need to be trained in the administration of injections on their own using the right syringe and the right dose.

102. (D) All of the above.

To determine the accuracy of medication orders for clients, things to be considered include the completion of the medical order, accuracy of the order, any client allergies, the health status of the client, and significant laboratory findings.

103. (A) 100% bioavailability and the swift onset of action.

Drugs taken intravenously have 100% bioavailability. This means that all the medication administered into the veins will reach the target organs. They are not subject to gut breakdown, which occurs in the oral route of administration. They are also very swift in action since they are able to enter the bloodstream in seconds to minutes. Intravenous administration is the route of choice in emergencies or when swift reactions are needed, e.g., in surgery.

104. (D) None of the above.

Routes of drug administration include oral, sublingual, topical, transdermal, inhalation, and intravenous.

105. (A) Cisplatin.

Cisplatin is a chemotherapy drug that is given intravenously only. Other drugs listed have other routes through which they can be administered.

106. (A) 14g, 16g.

The cannula sizes are designated in such a way that the largest sizes have the smaller number. Since this woman is losing blood, she needs large quantities of blood and fluid. Hence two large bore cannulas should be provided. Other smaller cannulas are used when a patient is to receive lesser quantities of fluids and for pediatric veins.

107. (C) Sublingual.

Nitroglycerin is administered via the sublingual route. It is placed under the tongue for a few minutes and the onset of action is in about one to three minutes. When absorbed, it causes dilatation, which leads to a decreased preload. It reduces blood pressure and also increases the heart rate.

108. (D) None of the above.

In illness management, the client must be given all necessary information, which includes treatable signs and symptoms of chronic diseases, the treatment procedures, and the financial cost of each treatment. Nurses should ensure to teach patients about home care strategies for their illnesses. The patients should also receive a follow-up schedule as part of the treatment plan.

109. (C) 4 g Mgso4—1 g Mgso4 per hour over 24 hrs.

The 4 g loading dose is given slowly as IV over 10–15 minutes. The maintenance dose is given as 5 g of Mgso4 put into 500 ml of normal saline to run for five hours. (1 g /100 ml/hour). This maintenance dose should be given continuously for 24 hours after the last convulsion or delivery of the fetus.

110. (B) 14 g Mgso4—5 g Mgso4 4 hrly.

The 14 g Mgso4 loading dose should be given as a 4 g IV (slowly over 10—15 minutes) and then 5 g into each buttock IM. The maintenance dose is 5 g of Mgso4, which is given IM into alternate buttocks every four hours. This maintenance dose should be given continuously for 24 hours after the last convulsion or delivery of the fetus.

111. (B) 1 mg IV bolus every 5 minutes.

When performing CPR for cardiac arrest adult patients, epinephrine (adrenaline) is usually given at a dose of 1 mg intravenously every 3-5 minutes.

112. (D) All of the above.

Administering anticonvulsants like benzodiazepines can help stop the seizure. Positioning the child on his or her side (usually the left to promote better heart function, but either side can be beneficial) helps keep the airway clear and prevents aspiration. Suctioning may be necessary if there's a risk of aspiration, especially if the child has secretions, vomit, or other obstructions in the mouth or airway.

113. (B) Chronic kidney disease.

CKD in the young presents this way. Kidney diseases are noted for facial swelling that is worse in the morning and regresses as the day goes by. CKD is also characterized by very high blood pressure readings in young people. Hypertension usually presents with just pedal edema, not facial swelling.

114. (C) Atrial fibrillation.

Atrial fibrillation is characterized by a rapid heartbeat that is irregular. It is usually detected first on examination when there is a significant deficit between the heart rate and the pulse rate.

115. (C) Asthma – Nebulize.

Classical signs of an asthmatic attack are wheezing, chest tightness, and difficulty breathing. The treatment is to nebulize the patient.

116. (D) A and B.

An unconscious patient might be suffering from hypoglycemia, and a dehydrated patient with ketone breath might be suffering from diabetic ketoacidosis (DKA). In the hypoglycemic patient, sugar might be low, usually values below 2.2 mmol/l, while in the DKA patient, blood glucose can be very high. RBG must be taken to confirm the diagnosis and determine treatment options.

117. (D) None of the above.

Findings of myocardial infarction on ECG include ST-segment elevation, T-wave inversion, hyperacute waves, Reciprocal ST depression, Q waves, and new left bundle branch block.

118. (C) Get informed consent.

Informed consent is the first step to take before running any test or procedures on the client. The informed consent should be written and signed by the client. The patient should be told the benefits, complications, side effects, alternatives, and health care personnel who will be carrying out the test.

119. (D) Mantoux test.

The Mantoux test is used to confirm the presence of mycobacterium tuberculosis in a patient. In the test, no blood is required. A small amount of tuberculin is injected into the skin, usually on the forearm. After 48 to 72 hours the site is checked to assess the reaction. A person who has been exposed to mycobacterium tuberculosis will mount an immune response that will result in an induration which is then measured. There will be no induration in a person who has not been exposed.

120. (B) To measure 24-hour protein.

The 24-hour urine sample is mostly used to measure the 24-hour protein, which is useful in the diagnosis of kidney diseases. It is also useful in pregnant women to test for preeclampsia.

121. (D) All of the above.

This patient is at risk of hemorrhagic shock due to blood loss. Hence, the bleeding should be stopped in any way possible, which includes sutures and packing. Blood can also be transfused if obtained immediately, and if not, volume expanders like ringer's lactate or normal saline can be used while blood is obtained for transfusion.

122. (C) A and B.

This patient needs to eat well so that the wound can heal well. When starvation occurs, the body slows processes down to conserve energy. There can also be a breakdown of body proteins if starvation is prolonged. The body's immune system is weak when a person is food deprived, so there is an increased risk of wound infection. There was no mention of diabetes in the condition of the woman; hence, there is no need to counsel her on it.

123. (D) A and C.

Normal hemostasis should occur in about two minutes or less if appropriate pressure is applied at the point of the venipuncture. However, if this is done and the bleeding does not stop for eight minutes, then it is possible the patient has a bleeding disorder that needs attention from physicians.

124. (D) A and C.

A patient with 80/50 mmhg of blood pressure is already hypotensive and will require some IV fluids to boost the blood pressure. While setting up the lines for the fluids, samples can be taken for further investigation. A fasting blood glucose might not be possible at this time, because the patient might have eaten and the time of the day is not conducive for the test.

125. (C) Pain.

Pain is a complication of surgery, but it can be managed with pain relievers. Osteomyelitis is the infection of the bone and it is one of the most worrisome complications of orthopedic surgery, as it can be very difficult to completely eradicate. Implants can also be dislodged.

126. (D) All of the above.

Offensive odors, pus from the wound, and fever are all signs of an infection. Others include breakdown of the wound, redness, pain, swelling, warmth of the site, or the presence of an abscess.

127. (A) Bell's Palsy, CN VII.

Cranial nerve VII is also known as the facial nerve, and it is responsible for the movement of many facial muscles. The affected patient cannot move a part of the face on one side or completely close the eye on the affected side. The patient might also be unable to hear well on the affected side. Bell's Palsy is the most common cause of unilateral facial paralysis. It usually resolves over time and the cause is unknown.

128. (B) Insulin.

Insulin is used in the management of hyperglycemia. However, it can also cause the patient to go into hypoglycemia if a very high dose is given or if the patient does not eat before taking the insulin injection.

129. (A) Educate and reassure the patient.

The role of the nurse here is to educate the patient on what would be done. Some patients also have worries, and the nurse should reassure them and address their concerns. Obtaining informed consent is usually the responsibility physicians or surgeons who will be performing the procedure, as they are best equipped to explain the risks.

130. (B) Headaches.

Headaches can result from spinal anesthesia. This is known as a post-spinal puncture headache, and it results from a drop in the CSF pressure if there is a leak through the puncture. Back pain might result from the puncture site, but it is less common.

131. (A) Ventricular hypertrophy.

Ventricular hypertrophy occurs when the heart, particularly the ventricles, continues to hypertrophy or increase in size to accommodate an increase in blood pressure. Atrial hypertrophy is not very common since the ventricles are the chambers that pump blood at the highest pressure. Atrial fibrillation is an irregular electrical impulse present in the atria.

132. (B) Kidneys.

The kidneys are the organs responsible for the removal of waste products from the blood through the ultrafiltration process in the glomerulus. When this process is affected, then there will be an accumulation of waste in the blood. The major waste product here is urea, which is a by-product of the breakdown of amino acids from proteins.

133. (A) Kernicterus.

Kernicterus, also known as bilirubin encephalopathy, refers to the brain damage that is sustained in the newborn from large deposits of indirect or unconjugated bilirubin in the blood. Normally, bilirubin is lipophilic and must be bound to albumin to get to the liver, where it is conjugated. However, if there is unconjugated albumin that is free, this can then cross the blood-brain barrier because it is lipophilic. Kernicterus causes hypotonia, poor feeding, and decreased alertness in the baby.

134. (A) It breaks down the bilirubin into soluble isomers.

Phototherapy works by breaking bilirubin down into photoisomers that are water-soluble and can be easily excreted via urine without liver conjugation. Phototherapy produces two types of isomers of bilirubin: structural (z-lumirubin) and configurational (4Z, 15 E-bilirubin) isomers. As this happens, the yellowing of the skin caused by bilirubin deposits is reduced and blood bilirubin levels begin to drop significantly.

135. (D) Skin infection.

A skin infection is typically not an indication for a central line placement.

136. (D) All of the above.

A patient who is moving cannot have a biopsy. A patient with an uncorrectable bleeding disorder can bleed as a complication of the disorder. When there is no safe path for the needle to pass through, a core needle biopsy is contraindicated.

137. (D) Post-oxygenation.

Post-oxygenation is not involved. Preoxygenation is the administration of oxygen before suction to maintain the airways. A sterile glove is worn, and the tip of the suction catheter is lubricated. The catheter is slowly advanced into the patient's airways to remove secretions from the airways. This process can be repeated until the airways are clear.

138. (D) Needle holder.

A needle holder is not typically needed for a wound dressing. A needle holder is more useful in suturing.

139. (D) Auscultation.

Auscultation is not involved in pulmonary hygiene. Pulmonary hygiene consists of simple and advanced techniques to clear the airways. The airway structures should be patent at all times so that air can flow in and out freely. Simple techniques include coughing, deep breathing and postural drainage. Advanced techniques include percussion and vibrations.

140. (A) Forearm/upper arm.

The forearm/upper arm is the preferred location for the AV fistula. An arteriovenous fistula (AV) is a connection between an artery and vein and is done three months before the dialysis to allow for maturity. The AV graft is preferred to the vascular access line because it stays longer and lowers the risk of infection.

141. (A) Administer IV Furosemide.

Furosemide is a diuretic. It is effective in pulmonary congestion, which is most likely what this patient has from heart failure from long-standing hypertension.

Other things can follow, such as oxygen, vitals monitoring, and samples for investigation. If the fluid in the lungs is not cleared, the oxygen saturation will not improve even when the patient is placed on 100% oxygen.

142. (B) Set up IV ringer's lactate.

This woman is hypotensive and dehydrated. She needs intravenous fluids first. When a line is set, samples can be taken to run other investigations. But ringer's lactate should be set up as a volume expander. From the results of the test and investigations, if hematocrit is low, then blood can be given to transfuse the patient.

143. (C) Tall Tented T-waves.

Other ECG features of hyperkalemia include Absent P waves, shortened QT interval, and depression of the ST segment.

144. (B) Pacemaker spikes.

Pacemaker spikes are the vertical signals seen on the ECG, which represent the electrical impulses that are generated by the pacemaker.

145. (D) Sinus node dysfunction.

Sinus node dysfunction is a class I and II indication for pacemaker insertion, depending on how it presents. All other answers listed are contraindications to the placement of a pacemaker.

146. (D) Asymptomatic bradycardia while sleeping.

Asymptomatic bradycardia while sleeping is a contraindication to the insertion of pacemakers. Acquired AV block is a class I and II indication. Symptomatic unresolving bradycardia is a Class I indication. Alternating bundle-branch block is a class I indication of insertion of a pacemaker.

147. (A) Device-related complications.

Device-related complications are most common within the first three to six months of discharge. Other common complications include hematoma, pneumothorax, heart failure, etc.

148. (D) All of the above.

A client must be educated about the etiology of the disease, the risk factors, pathophysiology and management or treatment. This helps to manage the expectations of the client, as well as provide a sense of trust and cooperation from the client. Patients tend to respond better when they understand what is being done.

149. (C) Spirometry.

Spirometry is a pulmonary function test that assesses the activity of the lungs, airways, and respiratory muscles by measuring the lung capacity, which is the total amount of air that is expelled from a lung filled with air. It also measures values like the maximal expiration, forced lung capacity and forced expiration value.

150. (C) A subacute condition is the same as an acute condition.

This is false. Subacute means it is rapid but not sudden. It falls somewhere between acute and chronic conditions. An acute condition can become subacute, and a chronic condition can also become subacute when exacerbated. An acute condition is a sudden, rapid health condition that requires an emergency response.

Made in the USA
Columbia, SC
21 December 2024